Must-Have Information for Pharmacists About Quality and Patient Safety

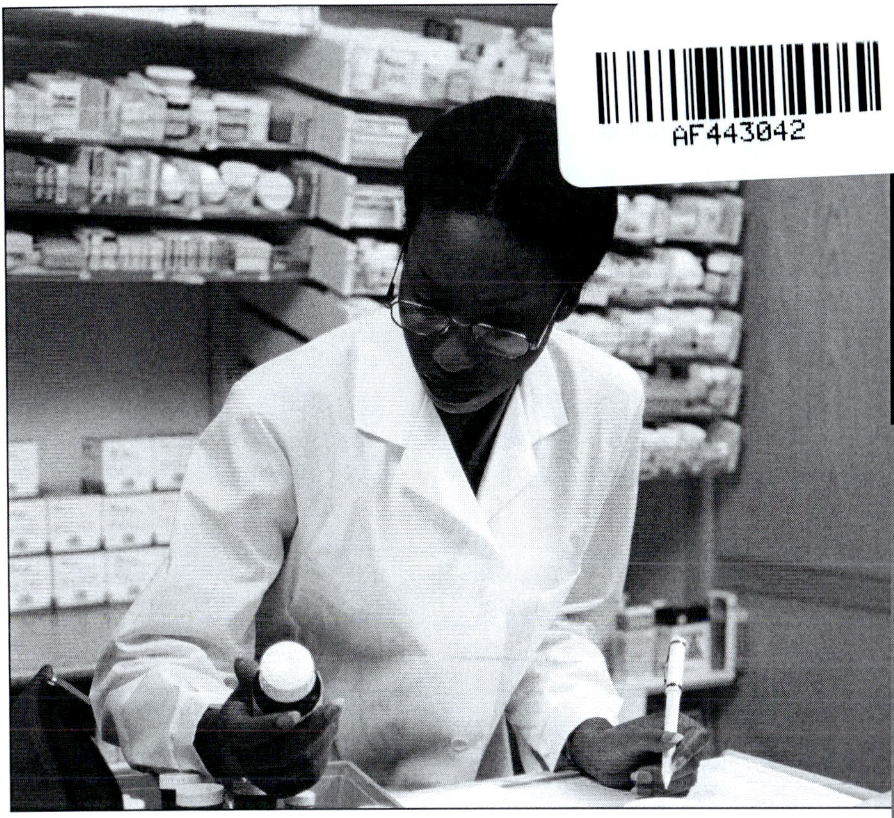

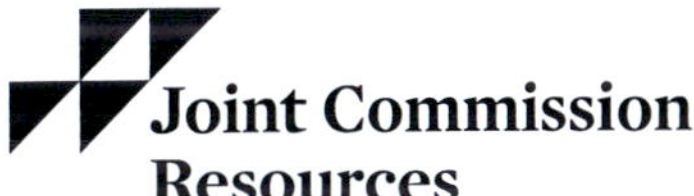

Joint Commission Resources

Foreword by
Philip J. Schneider, M.S.,
F.A.S.H.P., Clinical Professor
and Director, Latiolais
Leadership Program,
College of Pharmacy,
The Ohio State University

Senior Editor: Victoria Smith
Senior Project Manager: Cheryl Firestone
Manager, Publications: Diane Bell
Associate Director, Production: Johanna Harris
Associate Director, Editorial Development: Cecily Pew
Executive Director: Catherine Chopp Hinckley
Vice President, Learning: Charles Macfarlane, F.A.C.H.E.
Joint Commission/JCR Reviewers: Patricia Adamski, Peter Angood, Jeannell Mansur

Joint Commission Resources Mission
The mission of Joint Commission Resources is to continuously improve the safety and quality of care in the United States and in the international community through the provision of education and consultation services and international accreditation.

Joint Commission Resources educational programs and publications support, but are separate from, the accreditation activities of The Joint Commission. Attendees at Joint Commission Resources educational programs and purchasers of Joint Commission Resources publications receive no special consideration or treatment in, or confidential information about, the accreditation process.

The inclusion of an organization name, product, or service in a Joint Commission publication should not be construed as an endorsement of such organization, product, or services, nor is failure to include an organization name, product, or service to be construed as disapproval.

This publication is designed to provide accurate and authoritative information in regard to the subject matter covered. Every attempt has been made to ensure accuracy at the time of publication; however, please note that laws, regulations, and standards are subject to change. Please also note that some of the examples in this publication are specific to the laws and regulations of the locality of the facility. The information and examples in this publication are provided with the understanding that the publisher is not engaged in providing medical, legal, or other professional advice. If any such assistance is desired, the services of a competent professional person should be sought.

Printed in the U.S.A. 5 4 3 2 1

Requests for permission to make copies of any part of this work should be mailed to
Permissions Editor, Department of Publications
Joint Commission Resources
One Renaissance Boulevard
Oakbrook Terrace, Illinois 60181
permissions@jcrinc.com

ISBN: 978-1-59940-088-4
Library of Congress Control Number: 2007931796

For more information about Joint Commission Resources, please visit http://www.jcrinc.com.

Contents

Foreword

We Stand Ready

Becoming a Medication Safety Champion

One of the most challenging times in my life occurred following my term as Presidential Officer of the American Society of Health-System Pharmacists (1988–1989). Serving in the role was certainly a great honor and privilege, and it changed my life in ways that I could not have imagined. However, the opportunities that it opened for me following my term were just as unexpected. Because the role pulled me away from the hospital so much and for an extended period, my responsibilities had been reassigned to other staff members. Upon my return to the pharmacy department, no one was ready to give me back my responsibilities, and I felt as though I needed to carve out a new niche for myself.

During this time, I happened to attend a hospital board meeting where one of the board members, an important leader in the community, asked what we were doing to prevent patients from being harmed while they were at the hospital. We had just made a major change in the drug administration program, and he was concerned that the new processes might leave patients open to medication errors. As my responsibilities and role within the pharmacy department were somewhat undefined, all eyes turned toward me, and I was asked to "look into it."

Sixteen years later, my professional focus continues to be improving medication use systems. Within that time, patient safety and medication errors have become key issues for health care providers, and public awareness regarding these issues has increased significantly. After years of finding creative ways to cast our role as being something more than prudent purchasers and distributors of drugs, we pharmacists now have the imperative to take a more central role in improving the care of patients.

The Joint Commission's Role in Improving Patient Safety

Before the patient safety movement, I think it would be safe to say that everyone in the hospital, including pharmacists, dreaded a visit from The Joint Commission. Come survey time, it was "all hands on deck" to prepare documentation and ensure that all policies and procedures were current and in place. Back then, standards primarily focused on individual departments, and our records consisted of checklists that documented activities associated with quality of care. There was very little focus on actual systems or how departments and health care professionals worked together to treat patients.

Now, consider how much this has changed. The emphasis of standards today is on systems of care and how they are monitored and improved. If a serious error occurs, it is important and encouraged to show what has been learned, changed, and improved, rather than "circling the wagons" to avoid losing accreditation. The message and mission of The Joint Commission is now loud and clear: Health care professionals must work collaboratively to improve the systems of care, rather than independently to merely "keep their shop in order."

Pharmacists Help Reduce Medication Errors and Improve Patient Safety

Virtually every hospitalized patient receives medications, and medication use systems are interprofessional, involving at the very least physicians, pharmacists, and nurses who work together to make and properly implement treatment decisions that involve the use of medicines. Unfortunately, because so many people are involved, much can go wrong with this system. Sixteen years ago, a Harvard Medical Practice Study reported adverse medical events in 3.7% of hospitalizations.[1] "Drug complications" were noted as the most common type of adverse event (19%) followed by wound infections (14%).[2] These data suggest that of all systems that should be the focus of improvement, medication use should be at the top of the list. Today, although progress has been made, there is still a need to continue improving medication systems.

Errors resulting in "drug complications" happen at all steps of the process: prescribing, dispensing, administration, and monitoring.[3] To really improve medication safety, all health care professionals involved need to acknowledge that improvements need to be made and commit to making these improvements. Who will lead this effort?

Pharmacists come armed with extensive training in pharmacotherapy and the quantitative sciences, and they possess the skill sets and motivation to fill this gap. Just like I was asked to do 16 years ago, pharmacists can and will accept these responsibilities and can be patient safety champions for their organizations. We stand ready.

Philip J. Schneider, M.S., F.A.S.H.P.
Clinical Professor and Director
Latiolais Leadership Program
College of Pharmacy
The Ohio State University

References

1. Brennan T.A., et al.: Incidence of adverse events and negligence in hospitalized patients—Results of the Harvard Medical Practice Study I. *New Eng J Med* 327:370–376, 1991.
2. Leape L.L., et al.: The nature of adverse drug events in hospitalized patients—Results of the Harvard Medical Practice Study II. *New Eng J Med* 327:377–384, 1991.
3. Leape L.L., et al.: Systems analysis of adverse drug events. *JAMA* 274:35–43, 1995.

Introduction

Must-Have Information for Pharmacists About Quality and Patient Safety is a handy reference that provides student pharmacists with an introduction to the quality movement and a discussion of challenging quality and safety issues. The book also helps prospective pharmacists gain a better understanding of how they can contribute to a culture and environment where patient safety is a priority.

More specifically, Chapter 1, "Overview of Patient Safety Issues for Pharmacists," introduces student pharmacists to safety and quality challenges they will find in today's health care organizations. The explanations and tips are meant to give future pharmacists a road map of the key components of patient safety issues. The chapter also provides a brief background of the recent quality movement and identifies a few key players within the movement.

Chapter 2, "What Pharmacists Need to Know About The Joint Commission," introduces student pharmacists to The Joint Commission by providing a discussion of its mission, purpose, and safety initiatives. The chapter outlines the Joint Commission's National Patient Safety Goals, its survey process, the standards, and the accreditation process.

Chapter 3, "The Pharmacist's Role in Improving Quality and Patient Safety," examines the critical role that pharmacists play in improving quality and patient safety every day. The book even provides future pharmacists with practical advice for initiating and following techniques to enhance patient safety in all health care settings.

We hope this book will assist you, as a future pharmacist, to be more inclined to implement and adhere to quality and safety initiatives and be better prepared to assess and enhance the quality of care you provide throughout your career.

Acknowledgments

Joint Commission Resources wishes to thank Philip J. Schneider, M.S., F.A.S.H.P., Clinical Professor and Director of the Latiolais Leadership Program at the College of Pharmacy, The Ohio State University, for writing the foreword to this book.

We also wish to thank writer Dave Whitaker for his dedication and diligence in writing this book.

Chapter One

Overview of Patient Safety Issues for Pharmacists

As health care continues to evolve and expand, the individual roles and responsibilities within it also change, grow, shift, and advance. The role of the pharmacist, for example, has transformed from a medical support role to medication leader. Today, an increasing number of pharmacists participate in all aspects of the medication process—from collaborating with physicians on prescribing, preparing, and dispensing medications to providing information to nursing staff on how to safely administer medications and adequately monitor for adverse drug events (ADEs). Their efforts and expertise, as well as their active involvement in leadership decisions and interdisciplinary teams, can significantly impact an organization's efforts to increase patient safety.[1]

The ongoing examination of health care roles and the embrace of a collaborative approach to care are elements of a "quality movement" that for years has promoted improved care and safety within organizations. This chapter explores the current landscape of patient safety in health care, offering an overview of the industry's great strides and its many challenges. In order for individual health providers such as pharmacists to make a positive contribution toward improving quality and safety, they must first assess the issues affecting their own organization and the health care field in general. The pages ahead delve into these issues by doing the following:
- Profiling agencies and entities that continue to make a difference
- Reviewing the meaning and measurement of sentinel events and near misses
- Outlining vulnerabilities associated with medication errors
- Considering steps and strategies aligned with performance improvement

Supporting a Nationwide Focus on Quality

The quality of care delivered by health care organizations has long stirred debate among facilities, clinicians, insurers, patients, and others. In the 1990s this debate widened as health care costs skyrocketed, health systems merged and reorganized, reports of medical errors increased, and consumers became increasingly proactive in their care. Amid rising voices of concern for greater transparency and better reporting of performance levels in health care, many government and private entities worked to facilitate the sharing of performance data and to establish standards of care that would serve to educate both the field and the public.

In 1997 the formation of the President's Advisory Commission on Consumer Protection and Quality in the Health Care Industry signaled strong government support of this "quality movement" and its benefits to patients. Composed of 32 members representing consumers, health care workers and professionals, provider organizations, state and local government, and various health care experts, the commission was charged with advising the president about changes occurring in the industry and recommending ways to improve the quality of health care to protect patients and health care workers. The consensus report published by the commission in 1998 included suggested steps to create a "national commitment to improving health care quality."[2] As a result, the National Quality Forum was formed.

National Quality Forum

The National Quality Forum (NQF), a not-for-profit membership organization, was created in 1999 to develop and implement a national strategy for health care quality measurement and reporting. Its members are drawn from all areas of the health care field—including providers, insurers, employers, consumer groups, professional associations, accrediting bodies, researchers, and labor unions. NQF endorses quality measures for national use and promotes the use of evidence-based quality information to develop preferred practices for all types of health care settings.

One of the NQF's many projects—which have addressed topics ranging from performance measures for cardiac surgery, diabetes, and ambulatory care to preferred practices for palliative and hospice care—includes Safe Practices for Better Healthcare, a 2003 endorsement of a set of 30 safe practices (or voluntary consensus standards) that clinical care settings can use to reduce the risk of harm to patients.[3] For more information about the 30 safe practices list, applicable care settings for each practice, detailed specifications, and additional material, visit http://www.qualityforum.org.

In February 2006 NQF merged with the National Committee for Quality Health Care (NCQHC), an organization of health industry leaders focused on quality improvement. The NQF's and the NCQHC's individual programs remain intact. More information about the new collaboration is available at http://www.qualityforum.org.

Institute of Medicine Reports

Another important organization at the forefront of improving quality and patient safety is the Institute of Medicine (IOM), an independent scientific adviser to policymakers, health professionals, health care businesses, and consumers, striving to improve health. Two reports issued by the IOM's Committee on the Quality of Health Care in America have greatly contributed to the quality movement in health care. In focusing attention on patient safety, the IOM's 1999 report, *To Err Is Human: Building a Safer Health System*, estimated that as many as 98,000 people die in hospitals every year as a result of preventable medical errors. The most common errors listed in the report included the following[4]:

- Adverse drug events
- Wrong-site surgery
- Suicides
- Restraint-related injuries and death
- Falls, burns, and pressure ulcers
- Mistaken patient identities

The report laid out a comprehensive strategy by which government, health care providers, industry, and consumers could reduce preventable medical adverse events and set a minimum goal of 50% reduction in errors during the succeeding five years.[4]

TIP: The only way to reduce errors is to change the systems and processes that breed them.[4,5]

A second IOM report, *Crossing the Quality Chasm: A New Health System for the 21st Century*, published in 2001, addressed restructuring the health care system as a whole—including delivery and payment mechanisms—to provide better patient care and make the best use of available resources.[5] Sidebar 1-1 on page 4 lists the six challenges identified in the report that health care organizations face to improve quality and patient safety.

The *Quality Chasm* report also included recommendations for bridging the "chasm" or gap between the existing and the ideal health care environment. The proposed changes were based on health care organizations meeting six "Aims for Improvement"[6]:

- Safety
- Effectiveness
- Patient-centeredness
- Timeliness
- Efficiency
- Equity

> # Sidebar 1-1. Six Challenges for Health Care Organizations
>
> 1. Redesigning care processes to better serve chronically ill patients across settings/clinicians and over time
> 2. Using information technology to automate clinical information and make it accessible to patients and clinicians
> 3. Managing the ever-increasing advances in methods/techniques and ensuring that health care professionals are competent to use them
> 4. Coordinating care across conditions, settings, and services over time
> 5. Working to build more effective multidisciplinary teams
> 6. Incorporating process and outcome measures into day-to-day activities
>
> **Source:** Institute of Medicine: *Crossing the Quality Chasm: A New Health System for the 21st Century.* Washington, DC: National Academy Press, 2001.

The IOM reports have become key publications in the quality and patient safety movement and continue to be an influence in the health care industry.

The Leapfrog Group

One of the recommendations given in the IOM's report *To Err Is Human* was for large companies to use employer purchasing power to promote advances in health care quality and safety. This provided a basis for the founding of the Leapfrog Group in late 2000. Composed of mainly Fortune 500 companies and other large private and public health care purchasers, the group's aim is to initiate improvements in the safety, quality, and affordability of health care by recognizing and rewarding providers who make significant strides in these areas:

- Coronary artery bypass graft
- Percutaneous coronary intervention
- Acute myocardial infarction
- Community-acquired pneumonia
- Deliveries/neonatal care

The Leapfrog Group participates in many initiatives with other organizations. The group's Hospital Quality and Safety Survey asks hospitals to voluntarily submit data on four quality/safety practices—computer physician order entry; evidence-based hospital referral; intensive care unit staffing by physicians experienced in critical care medicine; and the Leapfrog Safe Practices Score (based on NQF–endorsed safe practices).[7] More information about the Leapfrog Group can be found at http://www.leapfroggroup.org.

Institute for Healthcare Improvement

In December 2004 the Institute for Healthcare Improvement (IHI) introduced its own quality and safety initiative by launching the 100,000 Lives Campaign. In working with other organizations to disseminate improvement tools and support expertise throughout the United States, the initiative's goal was to save 100,000 lives by June 2006 by accelerating the pace of improvement in hospital care through the consistent implementation of proven lifesaving interventions. Many groups—including the Agency for Healthcare Research and Quality, American College of Physicians, American Medical Association, Centers for Medicare & Medicaid Services, The Joint Commission, National Association for Healthcare Quality, National Patient Safety Foundation, and Veterans Health Administration—endorsed the campaign.

Participating hospitals collected data on the interventions listed in Sidebar 1-2 (page 6) and submitted it to the IHI in April and May 2006. In June 2006 the IHI reported that results had far exceeded expectations. Instead of the original enrollment goal of 2,000 hospitals, the program included more than 3,000 hospitals. The hope of preventing 100,000 deaths was also surpassed; data showed that participating hospitals had collectively prevented an estimated 122,300 avoidable deaths.[8]

In maintaining and even broadening the gains that have been realized through the initiative's six interventions, the IHI is now asking hospitals to make improvements to protect patients from 5 million incidents of medical harm over a 24-month period, which will end on December 9, 2008. The IHI estimates that 15 million incidents of medical harm occur in U.S. hospitals each year for an estimated 37 million admissions in the United States each year. The 5 Million Lives Campaign, as the latest initiative is known, enrolls more hospitals and promotes the adoption of additional interventions, which are listed in Sidebar 1-3 on page 7. More information about the 5 Million Lives Campaign can be found at http://www.ihi.org.

National Patient Safety Foundation

The National Patient Safety Foundation (NPSF) is an independent, nonprofit organization created in 1997 that devotes itself to improving the safety of patients. The NPSF is trying to lead the health care industry's transition from a culture of blame to a culture of safety by identifying and creating a core body of knowledge, identifying pathways to apply the knowledge, developing and enhancing receptivity to

Sidebar 1-2. Six Interventions of the 100,000 Lives Campaign

1. Deploying rapid response teams, which enables staff at any level to call on a specialty team to examine a patient at the first sign of decline (with the team responding to the patient's needs in minutes rather than hours)

2. Delivering reliable, evidence-based care for acute myocardial infarction to prevent deaths from heart attacks

3. Preventing adverse drug events by implementing medication reconciliation practices—a formal process of identifying the most accurate list of all medications a patient is taking; comparing them with physicians' admission, transfer, and/or discharge orders; notifying the physician of discrepancies; documenting needed changes, and providing the patient a list of medications on discharge

4. Preventing central line infections by implementing a series of interdependent, scientifically grounded processes

5. Preventing surgical site infections by reducing risk factors and optimizing evidence-based processes of care

6. Preventing ventilator–associated pneumonia by implementing a series of interdependent, scientifically grounded processes

Source: Institute for Healthcare Improvement: *Press Release: IHI Announces That Hospitals Participating in 100,000 Lives Campaign Have Saved an Estimated 122,300 Lives.* Jun. 14, 2006. http://www.ihi.org/NR/rdonlyres/1C51BADE-0F7B-4932-A8C3-0FEFB654D747/ 0/UPDATED100kLivesCampaignJune14milestonepressrelease.pdf (accessed Jun. 26, 2007).

patient safety issues, and raising public awareness and fostering communication about patient safety. NPSF's efforts include sponsoring the Stand Up for Patient Safety program to help health care organizations launch and maintain patient safety initiatives and providing research grants to advance patient safety issues. More information about NPSF can be found at http://www.npsf.org.

The Institute for Safe Medication Practices

Since 1975, the Institute for Safe Medication Practices (ISMP) has been devoted to preventing medication errors and promoting safe medication use. This nonprofit

> # Sidebar 1-3. Interventions of the
> # 5 Million Lives Campaign
>
> 1. Preventing methicillin-resistant *Staphylococcus aureus* infection by reliably implementing scientifically proven infection control practices throughout the hospital
>
> 2. Reducing harm from high-alert medications, starting with a focus on anticoagulants, sedatives, narcotics; and insulin
>
> 3. Reducing surgical complications by reliably implementing the changes in care recommended by the Surgical Care Improvement Project
>
> 4. Preventing pressure ulcers by reliably using science-based guidelines for prevention of this serious and common complication
>
> 5. Delivering reliable, evidence-based care for congestive heart failure to reduce readmissions.
>
> **Source:** Institute for Healthcare Improvement: *Progress in the 5 Million Lives Campaign.* http://www.ihi.org/IHI/Programs/Campaign/ (accessed Jun. 26, 2007).

organization started a voluntary practitioner error-reporting program to learn why errors occurred and shared lessons learned with health care organizations across the country. ISMP's subsidiary, Medical Error-Recognition and Revision Strategies, works with pharmacists to prevent errors caused by confusing or misleading drug names, labels, and packaging. ISMP's other efforts include publishing newsletters to educate health care professionals and patients; developing high-alert drug lists, dangerous abbreviations lists, and other medication safety tools; and presenting conferences on medication use issues. More information about ISMP can be found at http://www.ismp.org.

Agency for Healthcare Research and Quality

The Agency for Healthcare Research and Quality (AHRQ) is a federal agency devoted to improving the quality, safety, and efficiency of health care. It first started in 1989 as the Agency for Health Care Policy and Research as part of the Department of Health and Human Services. It was reauthorized in 1999 under its current name to sponsor and conduct research that provides evidence-based information on health care issues so leaders can make informed decisions that improve health care services. Some of AHRQ's efforts include educating health care professionals about when and how errors occur, developing research to foster a national strategy to improve patient safety, and working with public- and private-sector partners to implement evidence-based approaches to improve patient safety. More information about AHRQ can be found at http://www.ahrq.gov.

Additional Organizations Involved in Patient Safety Initiatives

In addition to the groups mentioned above, there are many other organizations involved in driving and shaping patient safety initiatives. For instance, organizations such as the World Health Organization and the American Society of Health-System Pharmacists all work toward the common goal of improving patient safety nationwide and, in some cases, worldwide.

Examining Sentinel Events and Near Misses

With its mission to continuously improve the safety and quality of care provided to the public, The Joint Commission supports its provision of health care accreditation with related services that encourage performance improvement in health care organizations. Those many services include the maintenance of its Sentinel Event Database and the dissemination of its *Sentinel Event Alert* newsletter.

A *sentinel event* is an unexpected occurrence involving death or serious physical or psychological injury, or risk thereof. Sentinel events are not the same as medical errors. Sentinel events are not always caused by medical errors, and medical errors do not always result in sentinel events. The following are the most common types of sentinel events, in decreasing order of frequency[9]:

- Patient suicide
- Wrong-site surgery
- Operative and postoperative complications
- Medication errors
- Delay in treatment
- Patient fall

Sometimes errors that might threaten the life or function of a patient are caught and corrected before they reach the patient and cause any harm. This type of situation is considered a *near miss*, which is defined as any process variation that did not affect the patient's outcome, but for which a recurrence carries a significant chance of a serious adverse outcome.

Reporting and Investigating Medical Errors

As the landmark IOM reports concluded, most health care errors are due to faulty systems that either allow mistakes to occur or don't protect against them. To make their care and services as safe as possible, organizations depend on staff reports of errors that occur—whether they cause sentinel events or near misses—so that systems can be reviewed and revised as necessary. For example, many drug names have similar spellings and pronunciations but are used to treat completely different conditions. A process for receiving verbal orders that does not include a step in which the nurse or pharmacist taking the order reads back the complete medication order for verification may be setting the stage for a medication error.

The Joint Commission's Sentinel Event Policy specifies certain types of events that are "reviewable" by The Joint Commission when reported by a health care organization or another source. The policy encourages organizations to report sentinel events voluntarily. The sentinel events and identified root causes are entered into the Sentinel Event Database, which provides statistics that show causes, trends, settings, and outcomes.

When an error or event is reported, organizations need to identify what went wrong through a root cause analysis. This process helps staff examine a system's components, how they relate to each other, and at what point the system is failing. A team that performs a root cause analysis first determines exactly what occurred, then asks why it occurred (that is, what were the immediate events or factors that contributed to it). Next, team members look for the underlying causes of those immediate events or factors, probing through as many layers of the system as necessary to find the most basic cause(s).

TIP: As leaders, pharmacists play an important role in encouraging error reporting among staff and in participating in root cause analyses. Only after root causes have been identified can effective action be taken to prevent similar errors from recurring.

Creating a Culture of Safety

The examination and repair of faulty systems should not be limited to reactive situations in which an event has already occurred. Many proactive steps can be taken to help prevent errors from occurring—such as improving access to information, standardizing and simplifying processes, and providing appropriate training for staff. As many health care leaders have noted, reducing medication errors requires a system-based approach. In hospitals, such an approach encourages "nurses, pharmacists, and other care providers to collaborate on teams to provide system-oriented, evidence-based patient care to ensure the safe and effective use of medications."[10]

A team approach to patient safety requires strong communication and an organization that creates and promotes a culture of safety.

Improving Communication with Patients

Cultural, language, and communication barriers can lead to mutual misunderstandings between patients, their families, and health care providers, which in turn can result in events, errors, and process problems such as misunderstood orders, wrong or missed doses of medication, and disruption of care continuity from one setting to another. The risk of miscommunication and unsafe care is especially great for Americans with basic (29% of the population) to below basic (14% of the population) literacy skills and the additional 5% who are nonliterate in English.[11]

The Joint Commission's accreditation standards underscore patients' fundamental rights and need to receive oral and written information about their care in a way in which they can understand.[12] Health care organizations should make effective communication a priority to protect the safety of patients. They should know and reflect the communities they serve—not only the primary ethnic groups and languages that are represented, but the general literacy level of the community as well.

TIP: Pharmacists and other health professionals should use clear, plain language and should question patients to make sure communications are understood.

In recognition of the importance of effective communication in the delivery of care, interpersonal and communication skills are a required competency of medical residents under the Accreditation Council for Graduate Medical Education standards[13] and for maintenance of certification from the American Board of Medical Specialties.[14]

Improving Communication Among Staff

Efficient and effective communication among an organization's staff is vital to quality care and patient safety. In recent years, the transfer of knowledge between pharmacicts and other care providers has been viewed as particularly beneficial to care. With a foundational understanding of biomedical, pharmaceutical, socio-behavioral, and clinical sciences, as well as postdoctoral residency training and potential certification, the extensive knowledge and therapeutic practices that pharmacists bring to a medical team are only as strong as the relationships they form with their professional colleagues. Developing peer relationships with the medical staff and directors of other professional departments is key to gaining influence and providing leadership that contributes to an organization's patient safety goals.[15] In addition, building relationships with front-line staff such as nurses, technicians, and so on, is critical.

Understanding Performance Improvement

Traditional, hierarchical cultures tend to have punitive environments in which staff members are afraid to admit their own errors or to report someone else's error. However, a culture of safety and quality should be patient-centered and should focus on a proactive, multidisciplinary approach to continuously improve processes and prevent errors and adverse outcomes. It is in an open, nonpunitive culture in which performance improvement (PI) finds its effectiveness. As a methodology for examining and improving processes and systems within an organization, PI involves the following:

- Identifying an opportunity for improvement
- Collecting data on measures pertaining to the relevant process
- Analyzing those data
- Formulating a plan of action based on the results
- Implementing the plan
- Monitoring the level of improvement through further data collection and analysis

Performance measurement (PM), a component of PI, refers to the systematic collection of data over time (or at the same point in time) and includes the elements of choosing measures, setting performance goals, evaluating and comparing data, planning and implementing data collection, and organizing and presenting data so the results can be used to improve processes. Reports that staff members share pertaining to safety and quality issues—such as falls, restraint use, or surgical site infections—are the result of PM and contribute to the strides in PI.

Examining Areas of Concern

When it comes to patient safety, each organization must assess its vulnerabilities, based on the types and extent of services it offers and the patient populations it serves. Some issues of risk are fairly universal across organizations or a specific setting. For example, staffing shortages, medication management, and emergency management can be problematic for all settings along the continuum of care. All of these issues are frequent topics of PI activities and study.

Staffing Shortages

Effective staffing involves providing a sufficient number of appropriately skilled and competent staff to meet the needs of an organization's patients. When a facility is well staffed, it is more likely to see better outcomes, lower mortality rates, shorter lengths of stay, and reduced costs of care. Unfortunately, more and more organizations are finding it difficult to retain the staff their patients require.

In a 2003 survey conducted by the National Association of Drug Stores, it was reported that there were 5,499 employment vacancies among 24,396 chain drug stores nationwide.[16] Shortages are not limited to drug stores and hospitals. Long term care organizations, home care agencies, ambulatory, and behavioral health care facilities are also struggling with shortages of aides and assistants, technicians, nurses, and other staff. An extensive body of research strongly suggests that low staffing increases the risk of poor patient outcomes in hospitals, such as medication errors, health care–associated infections, and patient falls.[17,18]

In many organizations, individual roles are expanded to prevent deficiencies in patient care. In this environment, communication and collaboration are key. Increasingly, pharmacists and pharmacy technicians serve as mentors to other staff, a role that is now being recognized in training and education.

Recruiting new staff with the appropriate skill set is a challenging process, but the need to retain current staff is another—and one that is often overlooked. Health care organizations across the United States are implementing creative solutions, and many experts and panels are compiling "success stories" on a regional and national level.[19–21] A collaborative, team-based culture that emphasizes mutual respect and high-quality communication among nurses, physicians, pharmacists, and other staff can lead to improved productivity and job satisfaction.

Medication Management

Medication errors are near the top of every health care setting's problem list. As pharmacists well know, the process of medication management encompasses the key elements of selection, procurement, storage, prescribing/ordering, preparation, dispensing, administration, and monitoring. Glitches can surface at any point in the process—from incomplete or illegible orders to inaccurate labeling to incorrect dosage. Several factors have made medication management more difficult over the past few years:

- The huge increase in the number of new drugs on the market
- The treatment of patients with comorbidities by several physicians who do not communicate with each other about the medications they prescribe
- The use of mail-order pharmacies that provide neither personal communication with a pharmacist nor (in many cases) a double check of new medications against those already taken by the patient

- The overabundance and awareness of look-alike/sound-alike drugs that are used to treat very different conditions
- The use of herbal and other over-the-counter medications[22]
- The increasing number of drug shortages

Sharing information can help organizations identify possible causes and solutions for high-risk areas. The U.S. Pharmacopeia's MEDMARX® system is a national online database that aggregates hospital medication error data and disseminates it to participants. To encourage participation, all reports are anonymous and use a standardized format. Organizations that contribute to the database can access information about common types of errors and find examples of how other organizations have handled specific problems. MEDMARX allows users to review the causes and contributing factors associated with errors facilitywide, thereby identifying specific "problem-prone" systems or processes that may need changing.[23]

Medication therapy management. Medication therapy management (MTM) is a distinct service or group of services that optimize therapeutic outcomes for individual patients. It is a strategy of medication management approved by the Academy of Managed Care Pharmacy, the American Association of Colleges of Pharmacy, and the American College of Apothecaries, among other organizations, which involves a patient-centered approach to medication management. By encompassing a broad range of professional activities and responsibilities within the licensed pharmacist's scope of practice, and in considering the individual needs of a patient, these services can include the following[24]:
- Performing or obtaining necessary assessments of the patient's health status
- Formulating a medication treatment plan
- Selecting, initiating, notifying, or administering medication therapy
- Monitoring and evaluating the patient's response to therapy, including safety and effectiveness
- Performing a comprehensive medication review to identify, resolve, and prevent medication-related problems
- Documenting the care delivered and communicating essential information to the patient's other primary care providers
- Providing verbal and written education and training designed to enhance the patient's understanding and appropriate use of his or her medications
- Providing information, support services, and resources designed to enhance the patient's adherence to his or her therapeutic regimens
- Coordinating and integrating medication management therapy services within the broader health care management services provided to the patient

Medication reconciliation. One of the most problematic areas in medication use today centers on making sure that organizations have an accurate list of patients' current medications upon admission and that the list is updated during treatment and passed on to the next care setting, provider, or practitioner. Organizations develop the medication reconciliation process to obtain and document a complete list of each patient's home medications and then compare that list to the admission, transfer, or discharge orders.[25] Having this type of process in place can help prevent errors by ensuring that required home medications are continued while in the health care facility, contraindicated home medications are discontinued, discrepancies in dosages or routine are resolved, and missed or duplicate doses are avoided.

It is estimated that 46% of medication errors occur during the patient's admission to or discharge from a clinical unit and/or hospital.[26] Other studies have shown discrepancies in medication orders to be frequent and that as many as half of all hospital medication errors occur at the interfaces of care.[27,28]

TIP: Incorporating protocols and processes for reconciling medications at each intersection of a patient's care has been shown to significantly reduce medication errors and adverse drug events. [29–31]

The process of medication reconciliation is designed to promote communication and teamwork in order to prevent medication errors associated with patient hand offs. The Joint Commission mandates medication reconciliation at the time of hospitalization and discharge and addresses the issue in its National Patient Safety Goal 8, which will be outlined further in Chapter 3.

Adapting to Medicare Part D. With the introduction of the Medicare Part D prescription drug benefit, the nation's pharmacists are playing a broader and more meaningful role in the delivery of MTM services.[32] By helping beneficiaries transition to Medicare Part D, assisting patients in understanding the prescription drug benefit, and making decisions about drug plans, pharmacists play a vital role in the success of the program.[33]

Although challenges remain, pharmacy leaders agree that this new plan creates leadership opportunities for pharmacists and is a positive step forward for the profession.[3] In light of these new opportunities, pharmacists should take the lead or work with their team to ensure that their facility is meeting medication management standards as well as the Joint Commission's National Patient Safety Goals. Pharmacists should also ensure the following:

- That their facilities meet and continue to renew their own safety goals
- That pharmacists and pharmacy technicians are current with credentialing and clinical practice guidelines, as required
- That personnel throughout the organization share a clear understanding of roles and responsibilities in medication use safety

Medication management and technology. Another important issue in medication management is the use of various types of technology, including computerized prescriber order entry, electronic medical records, computerized decision support systems, smart pumps, computerized notification of critical test results, computerized ADE monitoring, robotics, and bar-coding technology. Making these and other tools available to staff can help improve communication, allow easier access to key drug information, provide calculation assistance for dosage, monitor patients' medication use for contraindications, and offer decision support to physicians in choosing medications. Of course, technology alone cannot prevent medication errors; the organization using it must integrate it into existing care processes that focus on safety and quality.[34]

Emergency Management

Health care organizations must prepare for every kind of emergency from natural disasters to fires and plane crashes. They need contingency plans for providing emergency care and procedures such as evacuation and decontamination. To develop a plan, all emergencies that could potentially occur within the community are identified. Next, leaders and staff must decide the likelihood of each possible event and the effect it would have on the organization and community. This process allows leaders to prioritize the emergency management plan and concentrate resources on the most likely and potentially serious events. The plan can then be tailored accordingly.

Many factors must be considered in planning for any emergency situation, including maintaining internal and external lines of communication, finding room for a large influx of patients, maintaining supply inventories, calling in extra staff, and providing transportation and food for patients and staff. Emergency planning often focuses on hospital emergency departments and trauma centers, but in a communitywide emergency, all health care organizations may be needed—whether to help with triage and urgent care of victims, provide nonurgent care to others, shelter community members or patients from other facilities who have been evacuated, or provide staff and/or supplies to other organizations.

Moving Toward Accreditation

When an organization understands the various external and internal factors that influence its ability to deliver safe, high-quality care to its patients, it is ready to explore health care accreditation. The following chapters provide an overview of The Joint Commission, its services, the value of accreditation, and the role of the pharmacist in quality and patient safety.

References

1. Horn E., Jacobi J.: The critical care clinical pharmacists: Evolution of an essential team member. *Crit Car Med* 34:S46–S51, 2006.

2. President's Advisory Commission on Consumer Protection and Quality in the Health Care Industry: *Advisory Commission's Final Report* (archive). http://www.hcqualitycommission.gov (accessed June 19, 2007).

3. The National Quality Forum (NQF): *Safe Practices for Better Healthcare: A Consensus Report.* Washington, DC: NQF, 2003.

4. Kohn K.T., Corrigan J.M., Donaldson M.S.: *To Err Is Human: Building a Safer Health System.* Washington, DC: National Academy Press, 1999.

5. Institute of Medicine: *Crossing the Quality Chasm: A New Health System for the 21st Century.* Washington, DC: National Academy Press, 2001.

6. Berwick D.M.: A user's manual for the IOM's "Quality Chasm" report. *Health Aff (Millwood)* 21:80–90, May–Jun. 2002.

7. The Leapfrog Group: *Fact Sheet.* http://www.leapfroggroup.org (accessed June 19, 2007).

8. Institute for Healthcare Improvement: *Press Release: IHI Announces That Hospitals Participating in 100,000 Lives Campaign Have Saved an Estimated 122,300 Lives.* Jun. 14, 2006. http://www.ihi.org/NR/rdonlyres/1C51BADE-0F7B-4932-A8C3-0FEFB654D747/0/UPDATED100kLivesCampaignJune14milestonepressrelease.pdf (accessed Dec. 18, 2006).

9. The Joint Commission: *The Joint Commission Sentinel Event Statistics—June 30, 2006.* http://www.jointcommission.org/SentinelEvents/Statistics/ (accessed Jan. 30, 2007).

10. Nurses and pharmacists partner for patient safety: Collaboration, teamwork emphasized. *Healthcare Benchmarks and Quality Improvement* pp. 92–93, Aug. 2003.

11. National Center for Education Statistics: *National Assessment of Adult Literacy (NAAL).* 2003. http://nces.ed.gov/NAAL/index.asp?file=AboutNAAL/WhatIsNAAL.asp&PageId=2 (accessed Jan. 26, 2007).

12. The Joint Commission Resources: *2007 Comprehensive Accreditation Manual for Hospitals: The Official Handbook.* Oakbrook Terrace, IL: The Joint Commission, 2006, Standard RI.2.100.

13. Accreditation Council for Graduate Medical Education: *General Competencies.* http://www.acgme.org/outcome/comp/compFull.asp#4 (accessed Jan. 26, 2007).

14. Nahrwold D.: The changing role of certification for physicians. *ABMS Reporter* 11, Spring 2002.

15. Zilz D., et al.: Leadership skills for a high-performance pharmacy practice. *Am J Health Syst Pharm* 61:2562–2574, 2004.

16. Knapp K.K., et al.: Update on the pharmacist shortage: National and state data through 2003. *Am J Health Syst Pharm* 62:492–499, Mar. 2005.

17. Clarke S.: Staffing the organization for excellence. In Joint Commission Resources: *From Front Office to Front Line: Essential Issues for Health Care Leaders.* Oakbrook Terrace, IL: The Joint Commission, 2005, pp. 113–144.

18. Rogers A.E., et al.: The working hours of hospital staff nurses and patient safety. *Health Aff (Millwood)* 23:202–212, Jul.–Aug. 2004.

19. American Hospital Association (AHA) Commission on Workforce for Hospitals and Health Systems: *In Our Hands: How Hospital Leaders Can Build a Thriving Workforce.* Chicago: AHA, Apr. 2002.

20. Pennsylvania Department of Health (PDH): *State Health Improvement Plan: White Paper on the Nurse Workforce in Pennsylvania.* Harrisburg, PA: PDH, Jun. 2004.

21. Joint Commission Resources: *Health Care at the Crossroads: Strategies for Addressing the Evolving Nursing Crisis.* Oakbrook Terrace, IL: The Joint Commission, 2002.

22. Joint Commission Resources: *Using Technology to Improve Medication Safety.* Oakbrook Terrace, IL: The Joint Commission, 2005.

23. Santell J.P.: Medication errors: Experience of the United States Pharmacopeia (USP). *Jt Comm J Qual Patient Saf* 31:114–119, Feb. 2005.

24. "Medication therapy management services: Definition and program criteria," 2004.

25. Joint Commission Resources: Tips for reconciling medications across the continuum. *The Source* 3:3–4, Apr. 2005.

26. Bates D.W., et al.: The costs of adverse drug events in hospitalized patients. Adverse Drug Events Prevention Study Group. *JAMA* 277:307–311, Jan. 22–29, 1997.

27. Marino B.L., et al.: Evaluating process changes in a pediatric hospital medication system. *Outcomes Manag* 6:10–15, Jan.–Mar. 2002.

28. Rozich J.D., et al.: Standardization as a mechanism to improve safety in health care. *Jt Comm J Qual Patient Saf* 30:5–14, Jan. 2004.

29. Joint Commission Resources: Reconciliation failures lead to medication errors. *Jt Comm J Qual Patient Saf* 32:225–229, Apr. 2006.

20. Pronovost P., et al.: Medication reconciliation: A practical tool to reduce the risk of medication errors. *J Crit Care* 18:201–205, Dec. 2003.

31. Whittington J., Cohen H.: OSF Healthcare's journey in patient safety. *Qual Manag Health Care* 13:53–59, Jan.–Mar. 2004.

32. Rankin K.: *Can Pharmacy Squeeze the Devil Out of the Medicare Part D Details? Pharmacy Times.* http://www.pharmacytimes.com/article.cfm?ID=2330 (accessed Feb. 16, 2007).

33. Texas Pharmacy Association: Medicare Part D: Pushing the profession of pharmacy forward. 2004.http://www.texaspharmacy.org/tpaweb/Professional/MedicareD_Challenges.cfm (accessed Feb. 15, 2007).

34. Kuperman G.J., Bates D.W.: Using information technology to improve health care quality and safety. In Joint Commission Resources: *From Front Office to Front Line: Essential Issues for Health Care Leaders.* Oakbrook Terrace, IL: Joint Commission on Accreditation of Healthcare Organizations, 2005, pp. 65–90.

Chapter Two

What Pharmacists Need to Know About The Joint Commission

As mentioned in Chapter 1, the mission of The Joint Commission is to continuously improve the safety and quality of care provided to the public through the provision of health care accreditation and related services that support performance improvement in health care organizations. This mission statement reflects the fundamental purposes set forth by the American College of Surgeons when it created its Hospital Standardization Program in 1917. It was that program that transitioned into the Joint Commission on Accreditation of Hospitals in 1951. In 1988 the corporate name was changed to the Joint Commission on Accreditation of Healthcare Organizations to reflect the expanded array of accreditation programs that then included hospices and long term care, ambulatory care, home care, managed care, and behavioral health care programs. In 2007 the name was shortened to The Joint Commission.

In subsequent years, The Joint Commission has expanded to include accreditation programs for clinical laboratories, critical access hospitals, and many others, as well as a broad spectrum of disease-specific care and other certification programs. In examining the role of accreditation standards and their impact on patient safety, outlining necessary steps of the accreditation process, and stressing the importance of information dissemination and performance measurement, this chapter offers an overview of the ways in which The Joint Commission continues to support health care professionals and organizations striving to provide safe, high-quality care to each and every patient they serve.

Supporting Accreditation Through Related Services

Accreditation is the principal set of services that distinguishes The Joint Commission from other organizations that promote continuous improvement in health care quality and patient safety. The Joint Commission evaluates and accredits more than 15,000 health care organizations and programs in the United States. Accreditation is provided for the following types of organizations:

- General, psychiatric, children's, and rehabilitation hospitals
- Critical access hospitals

- Medical equipment services, hospice services, and other home care organizations
- Nursing homes and other long term care facilities
- Behavioral health care organizations and addiction services
- Rehabilitation centers, group practices, office-based surgeries, and other ambulatory care providers
- Independent or freestanding laboratories

While the Joint Commission's own continuous improvement efforts have for the past two decades focused on its accreditation process, it has become apparent over this time that accreditation is a necessary but not wholly sufficient means for achieving the Joint Commission's mission. For this reason, the Joint Commission's portfolio of mission-related services has grown beyond accreditation to include the following:

- Performance measurement
- Patient safety
- Information dissemination
- Public policy initiatives

Through these services, The Joint Commission can help an organization strengthen community confidence in the quality and safety of its care, treatment, and services. In select states, meeting Joint Commission standards and goals may fulfill regulatory requirements. Simply participating in its supportive process, however, offers organizations the opportunity to gain a competitive edge in the marketplace. For example, The Joint Commission can help an organization improve its risk-management efforts and business operations through the sharing of best practices, and it can enhance staff education and staff recruitment through its professional advice and counsel.

Understanding the Purpose of Accreditation Standards

To be eligible to receive payments from Medicare—the federal program that provides health care benefits to more than 42 million elderly and disabled beneficiaries—hospitals must meet certain criteria established by federal law. The Centers for Medicare & Medicaid Services (CMS), the federal agency within the U.S. Department of Health and Human Services that administers Medicare, has established conditions of participation that hospitals must meet to be eligible to participate in the Medicare program. Hospitals that meet the Joint Commission's accreditation standards are deemed to meet the conditions to be eligible for Medicare payment. The Joint Commission's status as a hospital accrediting body was established by statute in 1965 and, consequently, can be changed only by Congress.

Accreditation and certification are also important because thorough and ongoing evaluation of processes and performance is the cornerstone for continuous improvement. The Joint Commission publishes standards for each type of organization it accredits or certifies. These standards address key functions within the organization and define the performance expectations, structures, and processes that must be present to ensure safe, high-quality care. Nearly half the standards directly address safety concerns, including: infection control, medication management, staffing and staff competency, fire safety, security, restraint and seclusion, emergency management, and surgery and anesthesia.

The Joint Commission develops its standards in consultation with health care experts, providers, measurement experts, purchasers, and consumers. The standards also cover specific issues such as the following:
- Implementing a patient safety program
- Responding to adverse events
- Proactively analyzing and redesigning systems to prevent harm
- Communicating all outcomes of care (good or bad) to the patient
- Medication management and safety

Providing Structure That Stresses Patient Safety

The overall goal of accreditation and performance measurement is to reduce the risks to patients and ensure that they receive safe, high-quality care. The Joint Commission has incorporated patient safety into all aspects of its accreditation process and activities to help organizations, in turn, incorporate patient safety into all of their improvement efforts. Sidebar 2-1 (page 22) discusses how The Joint Commission has expanded its mission internationally to become a global advocate of patient safety.

Sentinel Event Policy

The Joint Commission's Sentinel Event Policy, established in 1995, is designed to help organizations that experience serious adverse events in patient care to improve safety. As introduced in Chapter 1, the policy encourages voluntary reporting of sentinel events to The Joint Commission and requires that a root cause analysis be conducted for each of the "reviewable" events outlined in Sidebar 2-2 (page 23).

Sentinel events that are reported to The Joint Commission are included in its Sentinel Event Database. The Joint Commission publishes sentinel event statistics that can be accessed at http://www.jointcommission.org/SentinelEvents/Statistics/ and are organized by type of event, setting, reporting source, outcomes, self-reported events by year, and method for review of organization response. The information

Sidebar 2-1. Joint Commission International

The mission of Joint Commission International (JCI) is to continuously improve the safety and quality of care in the international community through the provision of education and consultation services and international accreditation. JCI was established in 1999 to respond to a growing demand worldwide for standards-based evaluation in health care. JCI's accreditation standards are the first and only international set of standards that apply to health care organizations worldwide while still accommodating cultural differences.

The purpose of JCI accreditation is to offer an objective process for evaluating health care organizations that is based on international standards. The goal of the accreditation is to stimulate and demonstrate continuous, sustained improvement in health care organizations by applying international consensus standards and indicators. The JCI accreditation process is designed to be valid, reliable, and objective while providing for cultural differences and needs across countries. For more information about JCI, visit http://www.jointcommissioninternational.com.

from this database can be used to study the underlying causes of events, share experiences with other health care organizations, and reduce the risk of future sentinel events.

Voluntary reporting of events has several advantages, including the following:
- Using the reporting system to contribute "lessons learned" that can be shared with other organizations experiencing similar events
- Sending a message to stakeholders that everything possible is being done to ensure that similar events are prevented
- Having consultation available from Joint Commission staff during root cause analysis and formation of an action plan

To raise the awareness of both the health care field and the federal government about sentinel events and the ways they may be prevented, The Joint Commission periodically publishes the *Sentinel Event Alert* newsletter, copies of which are accessible at http://www.jointcommission.org/SentinelEvents/SentinelEventAlert/. The issues covered in the newsletter are prompted by results from the database of reported inci-

Sidebar 2-2. Reviewable Sentinel Events

A *sentinel event* is an unexpected occurrence involving death or serious physical or psychological injury, or the risk thereof. *Serious injury* specifically includes loss of limb or function. The phrase "or the risk thereof" includes any process variation for which a recurrence would carry a significant chance of a serious adverse outcome.

A "reviewable" sentinel event includes the following:
- Suicide of any individual receiving care, treatment, or services in a staffed around-the-clock care setting or within 72 hours of discharge
- Unanticipated death of a full-term infant
- Abduction of any individual receiving care, treatment, or services
- Discharge of an infant to the wrong family
- Rape
- Hemolytic transfusion reaction involving the administration of blood or blood products having major blood group incompatibilities
- Surgery on the wrong individual or wrong body part
- Unintended retention of a foreign object in an individual after surgery or other procedures
- Severe neonatal hyperbilirubinemia (bilirubin > 30 milligrams/ deciliter)
- Prolonged fluoroscopy with a cumulative dose > 1,500 rads to a single field, or any delivery of radiotherapy to the wrong body region or at > 25% above the planned radiotherapy dose

dents, and the recommendations for reducing risks are taken from the experiences of actual organizations and advice from experts in the field. Recent topics have included blood transfusion errors, inpatient suicides, surgical fires, and high-alert medications.

National Patient Safety Goals

The Joint Commission developed its first set of National Patient Safety Goals in 2002. The goals were based on data obtained from the Joint Commission's Sentinel Event Database and recommended by a panel of patient safety experts. Each year, the Sentinel Event Advisory Group reviews a pool of evidence-based, cost-effective, and practical recommendations for addressing the most common and/or serious problems identified by sentinel event data. Although the first National Patient Safety Goals were applicable only to hospitals, goals have since been developed for each accreditation program. Each goal has specific requirements, and compliance with applicable requirements is required for accreditation. Table 2-1 (below) lists the National Patient Safety Goals for 2008 related to medication safety. National Patient Safety Goals are also outlined specifically for each accreditation program. Program-specific National Patient Safety Goals should be referenced whenever possible. The goals are updated each year and can be viewed at the Joint Commission's Web site, http://www.joint commission.org/PatientSafety/ NationalPatientSafetyGoals/.

Table 2-1. National Patient Safety Goals for 2008 that Relate to Medication Safety

Goal 1: Improve the accuracy of patient identification.
Requirement 1A Use at least two patient identifiers when providing care, treatment, or services.
Requirement 1B Prior to the start of any surgical or invasive procedure, conduct a final verification process (such as a "time out") to confirm the correct patient, procedure, and site, using active—not passive—communication techniques.

Goal 2: Improve the effectiveness of communication among caregivers.
Requirement 2A For verbal or telephone orders or for telephonic reporting of critical test results, verify the complete order or test result by having the person receiving the information record and "read-back" the complete order or test result.
Requirement 2B Standardize a list of abbreviations, acronyms, symbols, and dose designations that are not to be used throughout the organization.
Requirement 2C Measure, assess and, if appropriate, take action to improve the timeliness of reporting, and the timeliness of receipt by the responsible licensed caregiver, of critical tests and critical results and values.
Requirement 2E Implement a standardized approach to "hand-off" communications, including an opportunity to ask and respond to questions.

Goal 3: Improve the safety of using medications.
Requirement 3C Identify and, at a minimum, annually review a list of

(continued)

Table 2-1. National Patient Safety Goals for 2008 that Relate to Medication Safety (continued)

look-alike/sound-alike drugs used by the organization, and take action to prevent errors involving the interchange of these drugs.

Requirement 3D Label all medications, medication containers (for example, syringes, medicine cups, basins), or other solutions on and off the sterile field.

Requirement 3E Reduce the likelihood of patient harm associated with the use of anticoagulation therapy.

Goal 8: Accurately and completely reconcile medications across the continuum of care.

Requirement 8A There is a process for comparing the patient's current medications with those ordered for the patient while under the care of the organization.

Requirement 8B A complete list of the patient's medications is communicated to the next provider of service when a patient is referred or transferred to another setting, service, practitioner, or level of care within or outside the organization. The complete list of medications is also provided to the patient on discharge from the facility.

Goal 12: Implementation of applicable National Patient Safety Goals and associated requirements by components and practitioner sites.

Requirement 12A Inform and encourage components and practitioner sites to implement the applicable National Patient Safety Goals and associated requirements.

Goal 13: Encourage patients' active involvement in their own care as a patient safety strategy.

Requirement 13A Define and communicate the means for patients and their families to report concerns about safety and encourage them to do so.

Goal 15: The organization identifies safety risks inherent in its patient population.

Requirement 15A The organization identifies patients at risk for suicide.

Requirement 15B The organization identifies risks associated with long-term oxygen therapy such as home fires.

Office of Quality Monitoring

The Joint Commission relies on information from a variety of sources—including patients and families, government agencies, the public, an organization's staff, and the media—to reinforce its oversight efforts and improve the quality and safety of care in accredited organizations. Such information often comes in the form of complaints. The Office of Quality Monitoring, established in March 1999, provides everyone with an easy way to contact The Joint Commission about standards-related, quality-of-care issues that exist in accredited organizations. Common complaints deal with issues such as rights, care, safety, staffing, and medication use.

The Joint Commission encourages anyone who has safety or quality concerns or complaints to bring them to the attention of the health care organization's leaders first. This will often lead to more timely resolution of the matter. Incidents may be reported to the Office of Quality Monitoring by phone, mail, or e-mail. Because many people do not want to sign or give their names for fear of reprisals, the confidentiality of information provided by those calling or writing is strictly maintained. The office does not deal with billing, insurance, payment disputes, individual personnel or labor relations issues. More information can be found on the Joint Commission Web site at http://www.jointcommission.org/GeneralPublic/Complaint/.

Exploring the Accreditation Process

The Joint Commission's accreditation process has undergone significant changes during the past few years. Shifting its direction from survey preparation to continuous improvement, the process focuses on systems that are critical to patient safety and quality of care. It encourages organizations to use the standards as guidelines for day-to-day oversight of operations, and standards have been revised and streamlined to facilitate this endeavor. While a more detailed explanation of the accreditation process is provided in the accreditation or certification manual for each program, the following material includes key features of this process.

Periodic Performance Review

Accredited organizations must complete a Periodic Performance Review (PPR), or one of its three options, each year to assess their continuous monitoring and performance improvement activities. Using an online tool, each organization evaluates its compliance with all applicable standards, Accreditation Participation Requirements, and National Patient Safety Goals. If the organization identifies an area in need of improvement, it must develop a Plan of Action and identify the measures that it will use to confirm that the problem has been resolved. Depending on what PPR option the organization selects, Joint Commission staff must approve any Plans of Action, and surveyors will validate that the measures were implemented and effective at the next on-site survey.[1]

Priority Focus Process

The Priority Focus Process (PFP) uses an online tool to help focus survey activities on the issues that are most relevant to patient safety and quality of care at the organization being surveyed. Information from a variety of sources such as the organization's electronic application for accreditation, previous survey findings, performance measurement data, sentinel event reports (unless provided voluntarily), complaints made to the Joint Commission's Office of Quality Monitoring, and external organizations is integrated to identify the important clinical/service groups (CSGs) and priority focus areas (PFAs) for that organization.

CSGs define patient and/or service populations for which data can be collected; each accreditation program has its own list of CSGs. PFAs are processes, systems, and structures in a health care organization that significantly affect safety and/or the quality of care provided; a list of the PFAs and related subprocesses is provided in Table 2-2, pages 28–29.

A summary report listing an organization's top four or five CSGs and PFAs is made available to staff and leaders annually and at the time of the triennial survey. This report helps surveyors identify relevant standards that should be addressed on site, as well as patient populations that should be represented in tracer activities (described later). The PFP requirement does not apply to critical access hospitals.

Unannounced Surveys

In January 2006 The Joint Commission began conducting triennial surveys of accredited organizations on an unannounced basis. This change emphasizes the tenet that safe, high-quality care should be provided at all times, and organizations should not have to "ramp up" for an on-site survey. Staff members focus on their everyday processes rather than on making "quick fixes" to comply with standards just before a survey, and surveyors are able to observe care being provided under normal circumstances. The shift to unannounced surveys also provides accountability to the public and raises the degree of confidence they can have in accredited health care providers. If an organization has truly incorporated the standards into its systems, it will be in compliance no matter when the survey is conducted, and the public will be assured that safe, high-quality care is provided all the time.

Table 2-2. Priority Focus Area Categories and Subprocesses Related to Medication Safety

Assessment and Care/Services (not applicable to laboratories)
- Assessment
- Reassessment
- Planning of care, treatment, and/or services
- Provision of care, treatment, and/or services
- Discharge planning or discontinuation of services

Communication
- Patient and family education
- Provider and/or staff–patient communication
- Staff communication and collaboration
- Information dissemination
- Multidisciplinary teamwork

Credentialed Practitioners
- Assessing competency
- Credentialing
- Granting clinical privileges and peer review
- Continuing education and organizational orientation and training for licensed independent practitioners

Equipment Use
- Selection
- Maintenance strategies
- Periodic evaluation
- Orientation and training

Medication Management (not applicable to laboratories)
- Selection
- Procurement
- Storage
- Prescribing or ordering
- Preparation
- Dispensing
- Administration
- Monitoring

(continued)

Table 2-2. Priority Focus Area Categories and Subprocesses Related to Medication Safety (continued)

Orientation and Training
- Organizationwide orientation
- Departmental orientation
- Job-specific orientation
- Training and continuing or ongoing education

Rights and Ethics
- Patient rights
- Organization responsibility
- Consideration of patient
- Care sensitivity
- Informing of patients and/or families
- Organizational ethics pertaining to patient care

Quality Improvement Expertise and Activity
- Identifying issues and establishing priorities
- Developing measures
- Collecting data to evaluate status on outcomes, processes, or structures
- Analyzing and interpreting data
- Making and implementing recommendations
- Monitoring and sustaining performance improvement

Patient Safety
- Planning and designing services
- Directing services
- Integrating and coordinating services
- Reducing and preventing errors
- Using Sentinel Event Alerts
- Meeting National Patient Safety Goals
- Using clinical practice guidelines
- Actively involving patients in their care

Staffing
- Competency
- Skill mix
- Number of staff

Tracer Methodology

A majority of the on-site survey process is the use of tracer methodology, which assesses care, treatment, and services by following the actual care experiences of patients within the different areas of the health care organization. There are two types of tracers: individual and individual-based system.

In an individual tracer activity, the surveyor uses the organization's PFP information to identify specific patients and follow the care of those patients from admission through discharge or transfer. (For laboratories, patient samples are traced from physician order through notification and documentation.) Surveyors try to select patients who are in the organization's top CSGs, who cross programs and/or have received care in multiple areas (such as a nursing home resident who is admitted to a hospital and then transferred to a rehabilitation facility), and who have been in contact with areas related to the individual-based system topics (infection control, medication management, and data use). Viewing the organization's systems from the patient's perspective allows an evaluation of both the components of a system and how the different systems work together as a whole.

Individual-based system tracers focus on a specific system or process across the entire organization. The surveyor uses information obtained from individual tracers and discussions with staff members to trace one or more of the following "systems":
- *Data use,* which looks at how the organization collects, analyzes, and interprets data to improve patient safety and care
- *Infection control,* which focuses on the organization's processes for the prevention, control, and surveillance of infection
- *Medication management,* which explores the organization's medication processes and subprocesses from procurement to monitoring of effects, as well as potential risk points

Because errors are so prevalent when patients are handed off between programs, units, organizations, and individual practitioners, surveyors pay particular attention to how staff and processes interact and coordinate care.

Emphasizing the Importance of Information Dissemination

Transparency in reporting on health care organizations' performance is vital to giving consumers and employers the information they need to make informed decisions, to maintaining the trust of the public, and to motivating organizations to continuously push to achieve better safety and quality. The Joint Commission provides organization-specific performance information to the public via its Quality Check® Web site, http://www.qualitycheck.org. The site provides information on an organization's accreditation status, identifies any standards compliance problem areas, shows comparative performance data for core measures and National Patient Safety Goals, and lists distinctive organization achievements ("merit badges"). Quality Check allows users to search for organizations by name, geographic location, or type of services (such as acute care).

Much of the information available through Quality Check is also shown on an organization's Quality Report, which is sent after its triennial survey and details the facility's performance and how it compares to that of similar organizations. Such comparisons can help leaders identify where they may need to concentrate improvement efforts. This report is also evidence of Joint Commission accreditation, which can be used as a strong marketing tool to demonstrate the organization's commitment to and advances in safety and quality to patients, insurers, and others. A sample Quality Report is illustrated in Figure 2-1 on pages 32–33.

Incorporating Performance Measurement in Accreditation

One of the ways that performance measurement data are integrated into the accreditation process is through the ORYX® initiative, which began in 1997. A key component of this evolving project is the identification and use of "core measures"—standardized performance measures for specific conditions and populations with precisely defined data elements, calculation algorithms, and consistent data collection protocols. These measures are grouped into sets; approved measure sets cover acute myocardial infarction, community-acquired pneumonia, heart failure, pregnancy and related conditions, and surgical care. Other measure sets for sepsis, children's asthma care, hospital-based inpatient psychiatric services, diabetes care, pain management, nursing-sensitive care, and the prevention and care of venous thromboembolism are being developed and reviewed. The core measures can be found on the Joint Commission Web site, in the Performance Measurement Initiatives section, http://www.jointcommission.org/PerformanceMeasurement/PerformanceMeasurement/.

Hospitals are required to collect performance data quarterly on any three applicable measure sets and submit the data to a performance measurement system, or vendor, that has been approved by The Joint Commission for participation in the program. The vendor then collates the data and provides the organization and the Joint Commission with a summary report, which shows performance trends and patterns

Figure 2-1. Sample Quality Report

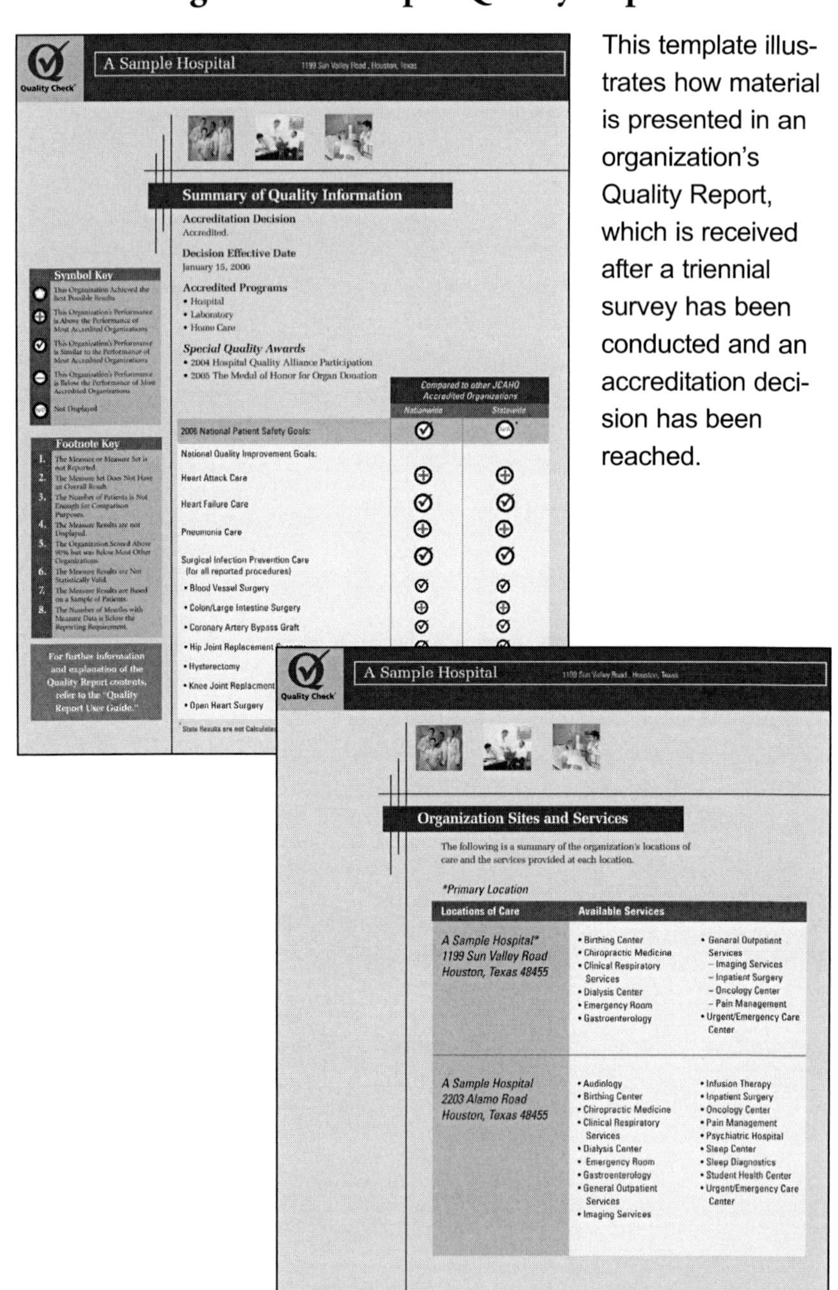

This template illustrates how material is presented in an organization's Quality Report, which is received after a triennial survey has been conducted and an accreditation decision has been reached.

Figure 2-1. Sample Quality Report (continued)

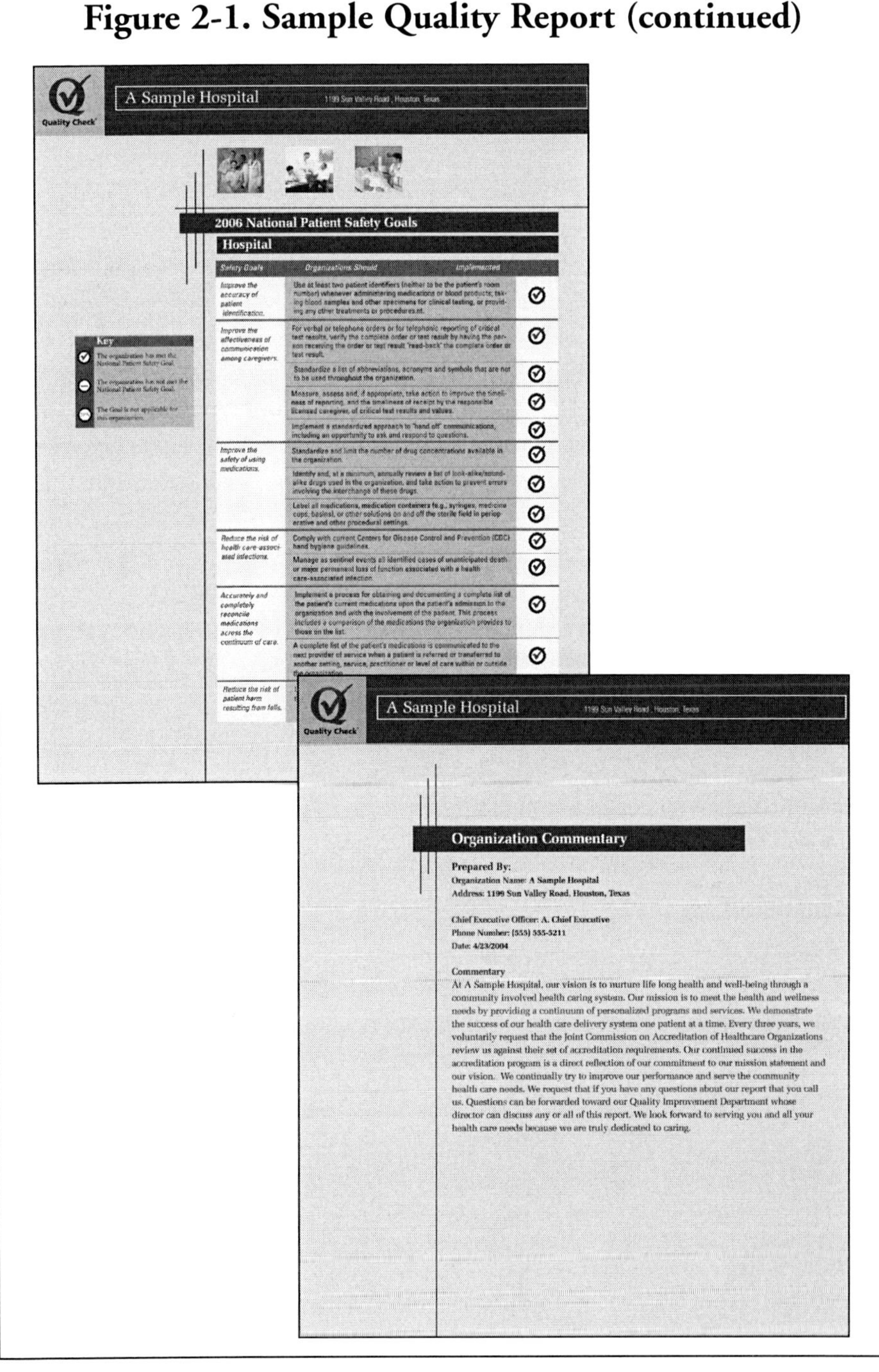

for the hospital over time and compares the hospital's performance to that of other organizations. Board members have probably seen these summary reports or highlights from them as part of regular improvement data reports. If a hospital's report shows a negative outlier (which indicates subpar performance) in a specific area for three or more quarters, the hospital must perform an analysis to determine whether a problem exists.

Participation in ORYX and core measure data collection is mandatory for hospitals. ORYX also includes performance measures (but not core measure sets) for behavioral health care organizations, home care organizations, and long term care organizations, which can choose to collect and submit data on a voluntary basis. However, home care and long term care organizations that participate in Medicare certification programs must meet the CMS requirements for submitting various forms of performance data. The Joint Commission plans to develop and gradually phase in core measure sets and requirements for all accreditation programs over time.

Also under development is a measure reserve library, which will provide health care organizations and other stakeholders with ready access to reliable, tested, and evidence-based measures that can be used to improve the safety and quality of health care. The basis for the library will be existing core measure sets (and new core measures as they become available). Over time, this will be expanded to include externally developed measures that have been evaluated by the Joint Commission against strict criteria. Each measure will include calculation algorithms and relevant data element definitions, and all sets will be submitted to the National Quality Forum for consideration and potential endorsement.

Establishing Priorities Through Public Policy Initiatives

Some quality- and safety-related problems pervade the entire health care industry and are simply too large to be addressed by individual standards or measures. For this reason, the Joint Commission decided to gather interested parties together and examine high-priority problem areas to develop and eventually guide the implementation of specific recommendations to resolve them. Initiatives usually involve the convening of an expert roundtable, the holding of a national summit, the issuance of an authoritative white paper, and the determination and implementation of appropriate follow-up strategies.

The Joint Commission's first public policy initiative, a major study on the nurse staffing crisis, was launched in 2001. Since then, other initiatives have addressed a

host of far-reaching topics:
- Emergency department overcrowding
- Emergency preparedness
- Health care professional education
- Health literacy and patient safety
- Hospital of the future
- Organ donation
- Pay-for-performance
- Tort resolution and injury prevention

The white papers from these initiatives, as well as additional guidance and educational materials, are available at http://www.jointcommission.org. Organizations may find it helpful to review the recommendations and strategies for adoption or adaptation to their specific needs.

Equipped with an understanding of how the Joint Commission works with health care organizations to improve safety and quality of care, pharmacists are able to serve as leaders in applying improvement practices in their own facility or system. Chapter 3 looks more specifically at the ways in which pharmacists can rely on this knowledge as well as their professional expertise to help create a culture of safety and quality.

Reference

1. Joint Commission Resources: *2007 Comprehensive Accreditation Manual for Hospitals: The Official Handbook.* Oakbrook Terrace, IL: The Joint Commission, 2006, pp. ACC-15–ACC-19.

Chapter Three

The Pharmacist's Role in Improving Quality and Patient Safety

Pharmacists who serve in hospitals, ambulatory settings, retail pharmacies, and industry are increasingly looked to as experts in medication management. When these experts step forward as influential players in their organizations, their contributions result in better patient care, improved medication safety, and enhanced pharmacy productivity.[1] Coordinated care between physicians and pharmacists alone, according to some studies, can improve patient care outcomes.[2–8] When their highly specialized knowledge and skills are integrated in a multidisciplinary team approach, pharmacists can positively affect economic and humanistic outcomes of patients as well.[9] Increasingly, managed health care systems and payers recognize that pharmacists—delivering consistent, effective cognitive services—improve patient outcomes and significantly reduce health care costs.[10]

Correcting and clarifying orders, providing drug information, suggesting alternative therapies, identifying drug interactions, and conducting therapeutic drug monitoring are among the many pharmacist interventions that can improve the safety and quality of health care provisions.[9] This chapter takes a broader look at the strategies and approaches pharmacists should consider for achieving greater results in improving patient safety. Relative to this pursuit, it also explores the pharmacist's role in the Joint Commission's National Patient Safety Goals and its Priority Focus Process. Additionally, this chapter stresses the importance of ongoing professional development for pharmacists.

Strategies for Improving Patient Safety

As pharmacists continue to emerge as leaders in medication management, their contribution toward improving patient safety increasingly includes putting their specialized skills to work in assessing and evaluating the processes in their department and their facility as a whole. By providing leadership in the drug formulary system, developing patient assessment skills, and participating in medical rounds and medication reconciliation, pharmacists can use their roles to make improvements in patient safety. In addition, in evaluating processes and in communicating issues and concerns with physicians, nursing staff, and other care providers, clinical pharmacists

are able to gather and share best practices systemwide and help ensure the following:
- That their facilities meet and continue to renew their own patient safety goals
- That staff members are current with credentialing and clinical practice guidelines
- That personnel throughout a facility share a clear understanding of roles and responsibilities in medication use safety

Whether or not their responsibilities are formalized by serving as a medication safety coordinator in their organization, pharmacists should play a proactive role in assessing and overseeing medication safety throughout the health care setting and initiate system improvements such as implementing changes designed to prevent mix-ups from look-alike and sound-alike drugs or installing a bar-coding system to verify correct medication dispensed to the patient.[11]

Providing Leadership in the Drug Formulary System

In the drug formulary system, pharmacists are essential participants in the process of establishing policies and procedures designed to educate and inform health care providers about drug products, usage, and committee decisions. The *drug formulary system* is an ongoing process whereby a health care organization, through its physicians, pharmacists, and other health care professionals, establishes policies on the use of drug products and therapies, and identifies drug products and therapies that are the most medically appropriate and cost-effective to best serve the health interests of a given patient population. A *drug formulary* is a continually updated list of medications and related information, representing the clinical judgment of physicians, pharmacists, and other experts in the diagnosis and/or treatment of disease and promotion of health. A *pharmacy and therapeutics* (P&T) *committee*, or equivalent body, is the mechanism for administering the formulary system, which includes developing and maintaining the formulary and establishing and implementing policies on the use of drug products.[12]

Along with pharmacists, P&T committees are comprised of primary care and specialty physicians and other health care professionals. Keeping in mind the multiplicity of drugs on the market and the continuous introduction of new drugs into the market, these committees meet regularly in order to keep a formulary current. P&T committees review monographs based on clinical literature that documents the following[13]:
- Clinical trials
- Relevant patient utilization and experience
- Current therapeutic guidelines and the need for revised or new guidelines
- Economic data

- Provider recommendations
- The safest, most effective drugs that will produce the desired goals of therapy at the most reasonable cost to the health care system

Pharmacists should analyze the formulary to remove dangerous drugs, automatically substitute safer drugs, and stay aware of drugs less prone to error.[14] They should also take a proactive approach in informing practitioners about changes to the formulary or to other pharmaceutical management procedures. They should initiate and oversee educational programs for payers, practitioners, and patients concerning roles and responsibilities and factors that affect formulary system decisions.

In any health care setting, a pharmacist should review every medication order to ensure the appropriate selection of drug, as well as the dose, route, and frequency. A pharmacist should also check for interactions with other medications. Depending on the setting, pharmacists can conduct the reviews either in the pharmacy or on patient care units if they have access to patients' profile information.[15]

Developing Patient Assessment Skills

In their efforts to improve patient safety, pharmacists should continually develop and sharpen patient assessment skills, including those of primary care patient interviews and physical examinations. In building procedural partnerships with leaders of other departments, they can create a reliable flow of assessment information to relevant care providers.

Pharmacists in the community setting have used their skills in patient assessment for years in dispensing over-the-counter products. They are well positioned to identify those at risk of cardiovascular disease, as well as undertreated patients at the point of dispensing. They also have an opportunity to identify at-risk patients based on their knowledge of a patient's family, what drug treatments are being taken, and other information that can be fed back to other care providers. Thorough communication of this information relies on the efficient design of standards and procedures.[16]

Pharmacists in a clinical setting use assessment skills to gather important clinical data that may aid in referral, treatment, or other primary care pathways. When a patient presents to the pharmacist with sudden symptoms of hypoglycemia, for example, patient interview skills, a general survey, and a limited physical examination may be used to obtain a clinical picture of the illness. In turn, the pharmacist may make an initial judgment on the patient's condition that may require immediate referral and/or treatment.[17]

In conducting patient assessments, pharmacists often employ a simple interview known as the "Basic Seven," an open-ended line of questioning designed to elicit a more detailed explanation. These questions, which are listed below in Table 3-1, can help the pharmacist determine whether or not to proceed with more steps, such as obtaining history, a review of systems, a general survey, or a physical examination.

Table 3-1. The "Basic Seven" Questions in Patient Assessment

Location	Where is the symptom?
Quality	What is it like?
Quantity	How severe is it?
	How does it interfere with the patient's life?
Timing	How long has it been present?
	When did it start? How often does it occur?
Setting	How did this happen? What was the patient doing?
Modifying factors	What makes it better? What makes it worse?
Associated symptoms	What other occurrences have taken place?

Source: Gilberson S., Stein E.: *Performing Patient Assessment: A Pharmacy Perspective.* http://www.fdlrez.com/HumanServices/pharmacy/pub2.pdf (accessed Mar. 6, 2007).

Participating in Medical Rounds and Medication Reconciliation

One of the most important steps in ensuring safe, high-quality care is enhanced collaboration among nurses, pharmacists, and physicians. In strengthening the relationships and protocols in the medication use system in a hospital setting, many organizations have included pharmacists on the medical rounds team. Their increased participation on medical rounds in many hospitals has been proven to prevent errors, lower drug costs, and reduce adverse drug events in intensive care units (ICUs) and medicine units.[5,18] A 1999 study by Leape and colleagues noted significant medication error reduction (66%) achieved by pharmacist participation on an ICU patient care team. Physicians accepted nearly all (99%) of the pharmacist recommendations tracked in the study.[5]

While their inclusion on the medical rounds team enhances the pharmacist's ability to oversee the quality of the entire drug distribution chain—from prescribing, drug choice, dispensing, and preparation to the administration of drugs[19]—it is through medication reconciliation that their expert oversight stretches across the continuum of care. Medication reconciliation can help prevent medical errors that include those associated with failure to continue needed home medications while in the hospital, failure to discontinue contraindicated home medications, failure to resolve discrepancies in dosages or route, and missed or duplicate doses resulting from inadequate records of frequent and last administration at transfer.

It is estimated that 46% of medication errors occur during the patient's admission to or discharge from a clinical unit and/or hospital.[20] Other studies have shown discrepancies in medication orders to be frequent and that as many as half of all hospital medication errors occur at the interfaces of care.[21,22]

Organizations have developed varying but similar definitions for medication reconciliation. In general, the activity is described as "a process for obtaining and documenting a complete and accurate list of a patient's current medications upon admission and comparing this list to the physician's admission, transfer, and/or discharge orders to identify and resolve discrepancies."[23]

Medication reconciliation involves a three-step process that entails the following:
1. Creating the most complete and accurate list possible of all preadmission medications for each patient
2. Using that list when writing medication orders
3. Comparing the list against the physician's admission, transfer, and/or discharge orders, identifying and bringing any discrepancies to the attention of the physician, and, if appropriate, making changes to the orders. Any resulting changes in orders are documented.

Incorporating protocols and processes for reconciling medications at each intersection of a patient's care has been shown to significantly reduce both medication errors and adverse drug events.[22,24,25]

The Pharmacist's Role in the Joint Commission's National Patient Safety Goals

As the process of medication reconciliation is designed to promote communication and teamwork in order to prevent medication errors associated with patient hand offs, The Joint Commission mandates medication reconciliation at the time of hospitalization and discharge and addresses the issue in its 2008 National Patient Safety Goal 8:

National Patient Safety Goal 8
Accurately and completely reconcile medications across the continuum of care.

Requirement 8A: There is a process for comparing the patient's current medications with those ordered for the patient while under the care of the organization.

Requirement 8B: A complete list of the patient's medications is communicated to the next provider of service when a patient is referred or transferred to another setting, service, practitioner, or level of care within or outside the organization. The complete list of medications is also provided to the patient on discharge from the facility. (Applicable to ambulatory care, assisted living, behavioral health care, critical access hospital, disease-specific care, home care, hospital, long term care, and office-based surgery.)

Any time a patient enters a health care organization where the patient's medications are relevant to the services provided or medications are to be ordered, this goal applies across the continuum of care. The ultimate responsibility for medication reconciliation lies with a prescriber, but the process should occur in an environment of shared accountability that depends on the expertise of the pharmacy.

The case example on page 43 illustrates the ways in which consistent meetings between department heads and other staff members can also be helpful in improving communication and care.

Improving Communication and Practices in Medication Administration

Pharmacists share responsibility in ensuring that an organization follows effective procedures in properly identifying its patients before medication is administered. The Joint Commission's National Patient Safety Goal 1—Improve the accuracy of patient identification—recommends that providers "use at least two patient identifiers (neither to be the patient's room number) whenever taking blood samples or administering medications or blood products. Acceptable identifiers may be the patient's name, an assigned identification number, telephone number, or other patient-specific identifier." The Joint Commission has subsequently determined that bar coding, including two or more patient-specific identifiers, will comply with this recommendation, which now provides organizations with another option for meeting this requirement.

National Patient Safety Goal 2—"Improve the effectiveness of communication

Case Example: Rural Hospital Runs on Effective Communication

Samuel Simmonds Memorial Hospital in Barrow, Alaska, is a 14-bed critical access hospital that relies on strong communication practices to ensure patient safety. The hospital serves 89,000 square miles in rural Alaska, and many of its patients are either treated and released or evacuated to other facilities, depending on their medical needs.

Due to the extent of patient turnaround at this facility, consistent and effective communication among all staff is essential to the tracking of and medical follow-up with patients. To this end, all oncoming physicians, as well as the clinical director and the director of nursing, meet with all on-call physicians every weekday morning to discuss the events from the previous night. In addition, on Tuesdays, the chief pharmacist, the dental director, the case manager, the medical records manager, the laboratory manager, and the radiology manager attend the morning meeting to receive patient updates.

Conducting these key meetings has confirmed to all staff members the importance of regular communication, as well as the positive impact resulting from the contribution of departments such as radiology and laboratory. Standardized communication between physicians and other key staff members has helped to ensure that everyone has adequate information to care for each patient.

Source: Samuel Simmonds Memorial Hospital holds meeting with on-call and primary physicians. In *Improving Hand-Off Communication.* Oakbrook Terrace, IL: Joint Commission Resources, 2007, pp. 91–92.

among caregivers"—is designed to ensure that the next care provider receives accurate information regarding the services, care, or treatment given to the patient. Pharmacists should recognize that communication of diagnostic imaging procedures and contrast media administration according to the facilities' processes are required to fulfill this goal.

Pharmacists should also be aware that National Patient Safety Goal 2, Requirement 2A, emphasizes the need for a "read-back" when verbal orders are received. According to this goal, the receiver should write down the complete order and then read it back to confirm the information given.

Table 3-2. The Joint Commission Official "Do Not Use" List of Abbreviations, Acronyms, and Symbols*

Do Not Use	Potential Problem	Use Instead
U (unit)	Mistaken for "0" (zero), the number "4" (four), or "cc"	Write "unit"
IU (International Unit)	Mistaken for IV (intravenous) or the number 10 (ten)	Write "International Unit"
Q.D., QD, q.d., qd (daily) Q.O.D., QOD, q.o.d., qod (every other day)	Mistaken for each other Period after the Q mistaken for "I" and the "O" mistaken for "I"	Write "daily" Write "every other day"
Trailing zero (X.0 mg)† Lack of leading zero (.X mg)	Decimal point is missed	Write X mg Write 0.X mg
MS MSO_4 and $MgSO_4$	Can mean morphine sulfate or magnesium sulfate Confused for one another	Write "morphine sulfate" Write "magnesium sulfate"

* Applies to all orders and all medication-related documentation that is handwritten (including free-text computer entry) or on preprinted forms.

† Exception: A "trailing zero" may be used only where required to demonstrate the level of precision of the value being reported, such as for laboratory results, imaging studies that report size of lesions, or catheter/tube sizes. It may not be used in medication orders or other medication-related documentation.

Requirement 2B addresses the use of inappropriate abbreviations. As shown above in Table 3-2, The Joint Commission has established an official "Do Not Use" list of dangerous abbreviations, acronyms, and symbols and requires each facility to add these to their own identified list. Pharmacists and other care providers should demonstrate caution when writing or giving verbal orders to ensure appropriate abbreviation use.

The Joint Commission's Medication Management (MM) Standard MM.4.10 requires medication evaluation by a pharmacist prior to dispensing for the appropriateness of the drug therapy and dosage, analysis of possible drug interactions, and determination of patient allergy history. "Pharmacists review each prescription or order for medication and contact the prescriber or orderer when questions arise (except when a licensed independent practitioner with appropriate clinical privileges controls prescription or ordering, preparation, and administration, as in endoscopy or cardiac catheterization laboratories, surgery, or during cardiorespiratory arrest, and for some urgent situations when the time to conduct a pharmacy review could harm the patient)."

The Joint Commission has also focused attention on this issue, with the addition of Requirement 3D to National Patient Safety Goal 3 in 2006, which states, "Label all medications, medication containers (for example, syringes, medicine cups, basins), or other solutions on and off the sterile field in perioperative and other procedural settings." See the full requirement, rationale, and implementation expectations in Sidebar 3-1 on pages 46–47.

Hospital inpatient pharmacies must have quality assurance programs in place when compounding sterile preparations to eliminate risks to patients.

TIP: Hospitals that outsource the compounding
of medications must be aware of
the conditions under which the preparations are compounded.[26]

In ensuring safe and effective medication therapy and optimal patient outcomes, pharmacists are also obliged to work with other team members to ensure that patients and their families understand their role on the patient care team. This corresponds with National Patient Safety Goal 13—Encourage patients' active involvement in their own care as a patient safety strategy.

At the outset of care, pharmacists can work with patients to develop a philosophy of ownership over the medical services they are provided. Pharmacists can establish a relationship in which patients look to them as a source for and as support in improving their own knowledge.

In the area of medication, pharmacists should encourage patients to take the initiative of understanding the methods and expected result of medications they are prescribed. Patients should know the following[27]:
- The name and description of their medication(s)
- The dosage, route of administration, and duration of their medication therapy
- The intended use and expected actions of their medication therapy
- Special directions and precautions for preparing, self-administering, or using the medication by the patient in the hospital or at home
- Action(s) to take in the event of a wrong or missed dose or interaction
- Significant side effects, interactions (including drug–drug interactions), or therapeutic contraindications that they may encounter and how to avoid and respond to such factors.

Sidebar 3-1. National Patient Safety Goal 3, Requirement 3D

Requirement 3D. Label all medications, medication containers (for example, syringes, medicine cups, basins), or other solutions on and off the sterile field in perioperative and other procedural settings.

Rationale: This risk reduction activity is consistent with safe medication practices and addresses a recognized risk point in the safe administration of medications in perioperative settings. Errors, sometimes tragic, have resulted from medications and other solutions removed from their original containers and placed into unlabeled containers. Medications or other solutions in unlabeled containers are unidentifiable. This unsafe practice neglects basic principles of medication management safety yet has been routine in many organizations with respect to medications transferred to the sterile field.

Implementation Expectations: Medications include any prescription medications; sample medications; herbal remedies; vitamins; nutriceuticals; over-the-counter drugs; vaccines; diagnostic and contrast agents used on or administered to persons to diagnose, treat, or prevent disease or other abnormal conditions; radioactive medications; respiratory therapy treatments; parenteral nutrition; blood derivatives; intravenous solutions (plain, with electrolytes and/or drugs); and any product designated by the Food and Drug Administration as a drug. Solutions include chemicals and reagents such as formaline, saline, sterile water, Lugol's solution, radiopaque dyes, glutaraldehyde, and chlorhexidine.

1. Medications and solutions both on and off the sterile field should be labeled even if there is only one medication being used.
2. Labeling occurs when any medication or solution is transferred from the original packaging to another container.
3. Labels include drug name, strength, amount (if not apparent from the container), expiration date when not used within 24 hours, and expiration time when expiration occurs in less than 24 hours.

(continued)

Sidebar 3-1. National Patient Safety Goal 3, Requirement 3D (continued)

4. Labels can be developed by the facility or commercially available; sterile labels can be purchased.
5. All labels are verified verbally and visually by two qualified individuals when the person preparing the medication is not the person administering the medication.
6. No more than one medication or solution is labeled at one time.
7. Any medications or solutions found unlabeled are immediately discarded.
8. All original containers from medications or solutions remain available for reference in the perioperative area until the conclusion of the procedure. All labeled containers on the sterile field are discarded at the conclusion of the procedure.
9. At shift change or break relief, all medications and solutions both on and off the sterile field and their labels are reviewed by entering and exiting personnel.

In March 2002 the Joint Commission, together with the Centers for Medicare & Medicaid Services, launched a national program to urge patients to take a role in preventing health care errors by becoming active, involved, and informed participants on the health care team. The Speak Up™ initiative is designed to increase patient involvement and communication with caregivers in order to reduce medical failures.

Brochures distributed to health care organizations, physician offices, and pharmacies and buttons and posters bearing the Speak Up slogan encourage patients and families to inform caregivers if they have questions or concerns about some aspect of care. More information about Speak Up is available at http://www.jointcommission.org/GeneralPublic/Speak+Up/.

The Pharmacist's Role in the Joint Commission's Priority Focus Process

Pharmacists can also impact patient safety through their participation in the Joint Commission's Priority Focus Process (PFP). While the PFP is a data-driven tool that helps focus survey activity on issues most relevant to patient safety and quality of care at the specific health care organization being surveyed, pharmacists and other care providers can use this framework as an instrument to prioritize improvement opportunities and maintain focus in areas of highest risk.

In focusing the surveyors' assessment on quality and safety issues specific to an individual health care organization, this process provides the organization with valuable insight on the priority focus areas (PFAs):

- Assessment and Care/Services (Analytical Procedures in laboratories)
- Communication
- Credentialed Practitioners
- Equipment Use
- Infection Control
- Information Management
- Medication Management (not applicable for laboratories)
- Organizational Structure
- Orientation and Training
- Rights and Ethics
- Physical Environment
- Quality Improvement Expertise and Activity
- Patient Safety
- Staffing

The PFP uses automation to gather presurvey data from multiple sources, including the Joint Commission, the health care organization, and other public sources. The PFP then applies rules to identify PFAs, relevant standards, and appropriate survey activities, and to guide the selection of patient tracers. The PFP does not imply that the PFAs are out of compliance or deficient in any way; rather, it lends consistency to the surveyor's on-site sampling process. By providing surveyors with presurvey information that has been developed using a standardized methodology, the PFP helps surveyors evaluate health care organizations' performance more consistently.

The output of the PFP includes the following:

- The top four-to-five *priority focus areas*—the processes, systems or structures within a health care organization known to significantly impact the safety and quality of care specific to the health care organization being surveyed
- The *clinical/service groups (CSGs)*—groups of patients, residents, or clients in distinct clinical populations for which data are collected. For example, in a hospital setting, CSGs might include cardiology, general surgery, or orthopedics and rehabilitation. In an ambulatory setting, an example of CSGs might be gastroenterology, obstetrics, and pediatrics.

Information from the PFAs and CSGs is then used to help guide the focus of the on-site survey activities.

Through the PFP, pharmacists can formulate improvements for their organization's own priorities by facilitating the following:

- Identifying their organization's high-volume and/or high-risk CSGs
- As part of standards compliance assessment, analyzing the systems or processes in these CSGs that are considered PFAs by The Joint Commission
- Analyzing the systems and relevant processes for any complaints or untoward events that have been reported to The Joint Commission

Given limited resources, all organizations must face the challenge of focusing their risk identification and reduction initiatives. Relying on the PFP to help guide an annual assessment process, organizations are better able to identify the year's priorities and develop procedures to deal with events that occur beyond priority areas.

Pursuing Ongoing Competence and Professional Development

With an enduring commitment to improve the quality of patient care, pharmacists in advanced clinical roles have in recent years shown increased interest in pursuing formal privileges and credentials to deliver specialized care.[28] The pharmacist's expanding patient-centered role, increasing specialization in pharmacy practice, and the need to document the pharmacist's ability to provide specialty care are also issues contributing to this positive shift. As the pharmacist's role continues to evolve, and medication use processes continue to adapt to clinical advances and new technologies, the benefits to safety and quality of care will depend on the ongoing professional development of pharmacists.

Continuing education in pharmacy has been defined as "a structured process of education designed or intended to support the continuous development of pharmacists to maintain and enhance their professional competence. Continuing education should promote problem solving and critical thinking and be applicable to the practice of pharmacy."[29]

In pharmacy, continuing education relates to professional development in the field as well as to the relevant competencies. Sidebar 3-2 on page 50 outlines the various pharmacy specialties recognized in credentialing and privileging.

Sidebar 3-2. Specialties Recognized by the Board of Pharmaceutical Specialties

Nuclear pharmacy seeks to improve and promote the public health through the safe and effective use of radioactive drugs for diagnosis and therapy.

Nutrition support pharmacy addresses the care of patients who receive specialized nutrition support, including parenteral and enteral nutrition.

Oncology pharmacy addresses the pharmaceutical care of patients with cancer and recommends, designs, implements, monitors, and modifies pharmacotherapeutic plans to optimize outcomes in patients with malignant diseases.

Pharmacotherapy is that area of pharmacy responsible for ensuring the safe, appropriate, and economical use of drugs in patient care.

Psychiatric pharmacy addresses the pharmaceutical care of patients with psychiatric disorders and is often responsible for optimizing drug treatment and patient care by conducting patient assessments, recommending appropriate treatment plans, monitoring patient response, and recognizing drug-induced problems.

Source: Board of Pharmaceutical Specialties: Current Specialties. http://www.bpsweb.org/03_Specialties_Current.html (accessed Jun. 10, 2007).

The Joint Commission standards require that the clinical privileges granted by an organization "fall within defined limits based upon the licensed independent practitioner's qualifications and current competence" and that consideration of initial, renewal, or revision of clinical privileges be based on peer evaluation of professional performance, judgment, and clinical and technical skills. The standards also stipulate that nonphysician providers may be appointed to the medical staff of the organization and granted clinical privileges if those privileges fall within the practitioner's scope of practice as defined by state law or regulation. The Joint Commission requires that "privileges awarded must be component specific and consistent with the organization's plan for service and its ability to support the care provided." In other words, competence to provide specific patient care services needs to be established locally by the health care organization, and not by a state board or other government agency.

The Joint Commission currently requires privileging for "licensed independent health care practitioners," defined as those who are permitted by law and regulation and by the health care organization to provide patient care without supervision or direction, within the scope of the individual's license and individually granted clinical privileges. It does not currently consider pharmacists to be independent health care practitioners, but this classification may change as the Joint Commission recognizes nurse practitioners and physician assistants as licensed independent practitioners where state law permits them to provide unsupervised patient care.

The education of a pharmacist is a continuum. One concept being discussed as a complement to pharmacist continuing education (CE) is referred to as continuing professional development and is based on a cycle in which individual practitioners reflect on their practice and assess their knowledge and skills, identify learning needs, create a personal learning plan, implement the learning plan, and evaluate the effectiveness of the educational interventions and the plan in relation to their practice. This ongoing, self-directed, and outcome-focused cycle of learning and personal improvement would augment CE offerings challenged to keep pace with a consistently changing and increasingly complex profession.[30]

As the profession continues to explore this and other improvements to CE for pharmacists, this statement by the American Society of Health-System Pharmacists continues to hold true:

> Next to integrity, competence is the first and most fundamental moral responsibility of all health professions. . . . Each of our professions must insist that competence will be reinforced through the years of practice. After the degree is conferred, continuing education is society's only real guarantee of the optimal quality of health care.[31]

References

1. Zilz D.A., et al.: Leadership skills for a high-performance pharmacy practice. *Am J Health Syst Pharm* 61:2562–2574, 2004.
2. Carter B.L., et al.: Interpreting the findings of the IMPROVE study. *Am J Health Syst Pharm* 58:1330–1337, 2001.
3. Chiquette E., et al.: Comparison of an anticoagulation clinic with usual medical care: Anticoagulation control, patient outcomes, and health care costs. *Arch Intern Med* 158:1641–1647, 1998.
4. Coast-Senior E.A., et al.: Management of patients with type 2 diabetes by pharmacists in primary care clinics. *Ann Pharmacother* 32:636–641, 1998.

5. Leape L.L., et al.: Pharmacist participation on physician rounds and adverse drug events in the intensive care unit. *JAMA* 282:267–270, 1999.

6. Gattis W.A., et al.: Reduction in heart failure events by the addition of a clinical pharmacist to the heart failure management team: Results of the Pharmacist in Heart Failure Assessment Recommendation and Monitoring (PHARM) Study. *Arch Intern Med* 159:1939–1945, 1999.

7. Bogden P.E., et al.: The physician and pharmacist team. An effective approach to cholesterol reduction. *J Gen Intern Med* 12(3):158–164, 1997.

8. Borenstein J.E., et al.: Physician-pharmacist comanagement of hypertension: A randomized, comparative trial. *Pharmacotherapy* 23:209–216, 2003.

9. Kane S,L,, et al.: The impact of critical care pharmacists on enhancing patient outcomes. *Intensive Care Med* 29(5):691–698, 2003.

10. The Academy of Managed Care Pharmacy: *Concepts in Managed Care Pharmacy.* http://www.amcp.org/data/nav_content/ Pharmacists%20Cognitive%20Services.pdf (accessed Apr. 3, 2007).

11. U.S. Office of Personnel Management: *Federal Employee Health Benefits: Kaiser Permanente Northwest Patient Safety Initiative.* http://www.opm.gov/insure/07/safety/57.asp (accessed Mar. 6, 2007).

12. Principles of a sound drug formulary system. *U.S. Pharmacist* 26. http://www.uspharmacist.com/oldformat.asp?url=newlook/files/Feat/sound.html& pub_id=8&article_id=652 (accessed Mar. 23, 2007).

13. Academy of Managed Care Pharmacy: *Information from the Academy of Managed Care Pharmacy to the Institute of Medicine Committee on the Assessment of the U.S. Drug Safety System.* Nov. 2005. http://www.amcp.org/data/legislative/analysis/AMCP%20info%20to%20IOM%20 Drug%20Safety%20Committee.pdf (accessed June 19, 2007).

14. Agency for Healthcare Research and Quality: *Beyond State Reporting: Medical Errors and Patient Safety Issues.* http://www.ahrq.gov/news/ulp/ptsafety/ptsafety9.htm (accessed Nov. 16, 2006).

15. Institute for Healthcare Improvement: *Improve Core Processes for Ordering Medications: Ensure Pharmacist Review of All Medication Orders.* http://www.ihi.org/IHI/Topics/PatientSafety/MedicationSystems/Changes/ IndividualChanges/Ensure+Pharmacist+Review+of+All+Medication+Orders.htm (accessed Mar. 7, 2007).

16. Petty D.: Drugs and professional interactions: The modern day pharmacist. *Heart* 89:ii31, 2003.

17. Gilberson S., Stein E.: *Performing Patient Assessment: A Pharmacy Perspective.* http://www.fdlrez.com/HumanServices/pharmacy/pub2.pdf (accessed Mar. 6, 2007).

18. Kucukarslan S., et al.: Pharmacist on rounding teams reduce preventable adverse drug events in hospital general medicine units. Arch Intern Med 163:2014–2018, 2003.

19. Kaboli P.J., McClimon B.J.: Clinical pharmacists and inpatient medical care: A systematic review. Arch Intern Med 66:955–964, May 8, 2006.

20. Bates D.W., et al.: The costs of adverse drug events in hospitalized patients. Adverse Drug Events Prevention Study Group. *JAMA* 277:307–311, Jan. 22–29, 1997.

21. Marino B.L., et al.: Evaluating process changes in a pediatric hospital medication system. *Outcomes Manag* 6:10–5, Jan.–Mar. 2002.

22. Rozich J.D., et al.: Standardization as a mechanism to improve safety in health care. *Jt Comm J Qual Patient Saf* 30:5–14, Jan. 2004.

23. Joint Commission Resources: Reconciliation failures lead to medication errors. *Jt Comm J Qual Patient Saf* 32:225–229, Apr. 2006.

24. Pronovost P., et al.: Medication reconciliation: A practical tool to reduce the risk of medication errors. *J Crit Care* 18:201–205, Dec. 2003.

25. Whittington J., Cohen H.: OSF Healthcare's journey in patient safety. *Qual Manag Health Care* 13:53–59, Jan.–Mar. 2004.

26. Newton D.W., Trissel L.A: *A Primer on USP Chapter <797> "Pharmaceutical Compounding–Sterile Preparations," and USP Process for Drug and Practice Standards.* http://www.nhianet.org/docs/usp_797_primer.pdf (accessed Dec. 3, 2006).

27. Joint Commission Resources: Performance improvement: Educating patients is key to safety. The *Joint Commission Perspectives on Patient Safety* 1:7, Nov. 2001.

28. Buckley B.: Privileging, credentialing poised for more growth. *Pharmacy Practice News.* June 2005. http://www.pharmacypracticenews.com (accessed Jul. 9, 2007).

29. Accreditation Council for Pharmacy Education: *Definition of Continuing Education.* 2003. http://www.acpe-accredit.org/pdf/CEDefinition04.pdf (accessed Apr. 10, 2007).

30. Rouse M.J.: Continuing professional development in pharmacy. *Am J Health Syst Pharm* 61:2069–2076, Oct., 2004.

31. American Society of Health-System Pharmacists. ASHP Statement on continuing education. *Am J Hosp Pharm* 47:1855, 1990.

Glossary of Joint Commission Terms

accreditation Determination by the Joint Commission's accrediting body that an eligible health care organization complies with applicable Joint Commission standards (*see* definition). *See also* accreditation decisions.

accreditation cycle A period of accreditation at the conclusion of which, accreditation expires unless a full survey is performed.

accreditation decisions Categories of accreditation that an organization can achieve based on a Joint Commission survey (see definition). These decision categories are as follows:

- **Accredited** The organization is in compliance with all standards at the time of the on-site survey or has successfully addressed all Requirements for Improvement (RFIs) (*see* definition) in an Evidence of Standards Compliance (ESC) report (*see* definition) within 45 days following the survey.

- **Provisional Accreditation** The organization fails to successfully address all RFIs in an ESC report within 45 days following the posting of the Accreditation Survey Findings Report (*see* definition).

- **Conditional Accreditation** The organization is not in substantial compliance with the standards, as usually evidenced by a count of the number of standards identified as not compliant at the time of survey, which is between 1½ and 3 standard deviations above the mean number of noncompliant standards for organizations in that accreditation program. The organization must remedy identified problem areas through preparation and submission of an ESC report and subsequently undergo an on-site, follow-up survey.

- **Preliminary Denial of Accreditation** There is a preliminary finding of justification to deny accreditation to the organization, as usually evidenced by a count of the number of noncompliant standards at the time of survey, which is at least three standard deviations above the mean number of standards identified as not compliant for organizations in that accreditation program. The decision is subject to review and appeal prior to the determination of a final denial of accreditation.

- **Denial of Accreditation** The organization has been denied accreditation. All review and appeal opportunities have been exhausted.

- **Preliminary Accreditation** The organization demonstrates compliance with selected standards in the first of two surveys conducted under the Early Survey Policy Option 1 (*see* definition).

accreditation process A continuous process whereby health care organizations are required to demonstrate to The Joint Commission that they are providing safe, high quality of care, as determined by compliance with Joint Commission standards, National Patient Safety Goals recommendations, and performance measurement requirements. Key components of this process are an on-site evaluation of an organization by Joint Commission surveyors, a Periodic Performance Review, and quarterly submission of performance measurement data to The Joint Commission, as applicable.

accreditation survey findings Findings from an on-site evaluation conducted by Joint Commission's surveyors that result in an organization's accreditation decision.

Accreditation Survey Findings Report A report of an organization's survey findings; the report includes requirements for improvement (see definition) and supplemental findings, as appropriate.

Accreditation *See* accreditation decisions

complex organization survey A Joint Commission survey in which standards from more than one accreditation manual are used in assessing compliance. This type of survey may include using specialist surveyors appropriate to the standards selected for survey.

compliance with a standard (*see* definition) Meeting the requirements of a standard through compliance with its element(s) of performance.

component A health care delivery entity (for example, service, program, related entity) that meets survey eligibility criteria under one of the Joint Commission accreditation programs. Multiple components comprise a complex organization.

Conditional Accreditation *See* accreditation decisions.

consultation 1. Provision of professional advice or services. 2. For purposes of Joint Commission accreditation, advice that is given to staff members of surveyed organizations relating to compliance with standards that are the subject of the survey.

criteria 1. Expected level(s) of achievement, or specifications against which performance or quality may be compared. 2. For purposes of eligibility for a Joint Commission survey, the conditions necessary for health care organizations and networks to be surveyed for accreditation by The Joint Commission.

Denial of Accreditation *See* accreditation decisions.

e-App The electronic version of an organization's application for accreditation.

Early Survey Policy A policy that provides two options to organizations undergoing their initial Joint Commission survey. Under both options, the organization undergoes two surveys. Under the first option, the first survey is limited in scope and successful completion results in Preliminary Accreditation (see definition). Under the second option, the first survey is a full survey, and successful completion can lead to the organization being Accredited (see definition). The second survey in both options is required and will address all standards and a 4-month track record of compliance with the standards.

Elements of Performance (EPs) The specific performance expectations and/or structures or processes that must be in place in order for an organization to provide safe, high-quality care, treatment, and services.

Evidence of Standards Compliance report (ESC) A report submitted by a surveyed organization within 45 days of its survey, which details the action(s) that it took to bring itself into compliance with a standard or clarifies why the organization believes that it was in compliance with the standard for which it received a requirement for improvement. An ESC report must address compliance at the element of performance (EP) level and include a measurement of success (MOS) (see definition) for all appropriate EP corrections.

The Joint Commission An independent, not-for-profit organization dedicated to improving the quality of care in organized health care settings. Founded in 1951, its members represent the American College of Physicians-American Society of Internal Medicine, the American College of Surgeons, the American Dental Association, the American Hospital Association, the American Medical Association, the public, and the nursing profession. The Joint Commission engages in issues and activities concerning the advancement of health care safety and quality, including public policy initiatives, standards development, and accreditation and certification programs.

measure of success (MOS) A numerical or quantifiable measure usually related to an audit that determines if an action was effective and sustained due four months after Evidence of Standards Compliance (see definition) approval.

National Patient Safety Goals A series of safety-related requirements developed by The Joint Commission that address the most common and/or serious problems identified by the organization's sentinel event data. The goals' applicability varies by accreditation program and all are reviewed annually for possible revision. Compliance with the goals is a part of the accreditation process.

near miss Used to describe any process variation which did not affect an outcome, but for which a recurrence carries a significant chance of a serious adverse outcome. Such a "near miss" falls within the scope of the definition of a sentinel event, but outside the scope of those sentinel events that are subject to review by The Joint Commission under its Sentinel Event Policy.

Periodic Performance Review (PPR) An additional requirement of the accreditation process whereby an organization reviews its compliance with all applicable Joint Commission standards, completes and submits to The Joint Commission a plan of action (see definition) for any standard not in full compliance, including the identification of a measure of success (MOS) (see definition), and chooses to engage in a telephone discussion with a member of the Standards Interpretation Group staff to determine the acceptability of the plan of action. The PPR will encourage organizations to be in continuous compliance with Joint Commission standards. At the time of the next full survey, surveyors will validate that the MOS(s) were implemented and effective.

plan of action A plan detailing the action(s) that an organization will take in order to come into compliance with a Joint Commission standard. A plan of action must be completed for each element of performance (EP) (see definition) associated with a noncompliant standard. A measure of success (MOS) (see definition) must also be included in the plan of action as indicated in the accreditation manual.

Preliminary Accreditation *See* accreditation decisions.

Preliminary Denial of Accreditation *See* accreditation decisions.

primary source verification Verification of an individual health care practitioner's reported qualifications by the original source or an approved agent of that source. Methods for conducting primary source verification of credentials include direct correspondence, documented telephone verification, or secure electronic verification from the original qualification source or reports from credentials verification organizations that meet the 10 Joint Commission requirements.

priority focus areas Processes, systems, or structures in a health care organization that significantly impact the quality and safety of care. The priority focus areas are

- Assessment and Care/Services
- Communication
- Credentialed Practitioners
- Equipment Use
- Infection Control
- Information Management
- Medication Management
- Organizational Structure
- Orientation and Training
- Patient Safety
- Physical Environment
- Quality Improvement Expertise and Activity
- Rights and Ethics
- Staffing

primary priority focus area Every standard is linked to one or more priority focus areas. When a surveyor has findings under a standard, he/she determines which of the linked priority focus areas is most related to the specific finding and this becomes the primary priority focus area. The organization's accreditation report is organized by priority focus area.

secondary priority focus areas The additional priority focus areas that are also related to a specific finding, in addition to the primary priority focus area. The organization's accreditation report also lists the secondary priority focus area(s).

priority focus process (PFP) The process for standardizing the priorities for sampling during an organization's survey based on information collected about the organization prior to survey. The process also helps to focus the survey on areas that are critical to that organization's patient safety and quality of care processes. Examples of such information may include, but are not limited to, data from the organization's e-App (see definition); compliance and sentinel event information; and data collected from external sources.

Priority Focus Tool An automated tool that supports the Priority Focus Process (see definition) through the use of algorithms, or sets of rules, to transform a health care organization's data into information that guides the survey process.

provisional accreditation *See* accreditation decisions.

Public Information Policy A Joint Commission policy governing the disclosure of specific information about the performance of a health care organization or network, as well as accreditation-related information that will remain confidential. This policy covers The Joint Commission's performance reports, information publicly disclosed on request, complaint information, aggregate performance data, data released to government agencies, and The Joint Commission's right to clarify information an accredited organization releases about its accreditation status.

Quality Report A report that is available to the public that provides information about an organization's accreditation decision and the effective date for the decision, any special quality awards the organization received, the accreditation services included in the organization's accreditation award, any disease-specific care certification(s) and the effective date of each certification received by the organization, the implementation of National Patient Safety Goals by the organization, the organization's performance against National Quality Goals and the organization's performance in relation to Patient Experience of Care measures.

requirement for improvement (RFI) A recommendation that is required to be addressed in an organization's Evidence of Standards Compliance (*see* definition), and needs to be addressed in order for the organization to retain its accreditation decision. Failure to adequately address a requirement for improvement after two opportunities will result in a recommendation to place the organization in Conditional Accreditation (*see* definition).

sentinel event An unexpected occurrence involving death or serious physical or psychological injury, or the risk thereof. Serious injury specifically includes loss of limb or function. The phrase "or the risk thereof" includes any process variation for which a recurrence would carry a significant chance of a serious adverse outcome.

standard A statement that defines the performance expectations, structures, or processes that must be in place for an organization to provide safe and high quality care, treatment, and service.

supplemental finding A recommendation that is not required to be addressed in an organization's Evidence of Standards Compliance (*see* definition), but should be addressed by the organization internally. A supplemental finding will also be factored into an organization's Priority Focus Process at its next survey.

survey A key component in the accreditation process, whereby a surveyor(s) conducts an on-site evaluation of an organization's compliance with Joint Commission standards.

full survey A survey that assesses an organization's compliance with all applicable Joint Commission standards.

initial survey A survey of a health care organization not previously accredited by the Joint Commission, or a survey of an organization performed without reference to any prior survey findings.

surveyor For purposes of Joint Commission accreditation, a physician, nurse, administrator, laboratorian, or any other health care professional who meets The Joint Commission's surveyor selection criteria, has passed the surveyor certification examination, evaluates standards compliance, and provides education and consultation regarding standards compliance to surveyed organizations or networks.

system tracer A session during the on-site survey devoted to evaluating high-priority safety and quality of care issues on a systemwide basis throughout the organization. Examples of such issues may include infection control, medication management, staffing effectiveness and the use of data.